An Atlas of
DIFFERENTIAL DIAGNOSIS
IN HIV DISEASE

Second edition

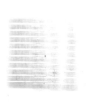

THE ENCYCLOPEDIA OF VISUAL MEDICINE SERIES

An Atlas of
DIFFERENTIAL DIAGNOSIS
IN HIV DISEASE

Second edition

M.C.I. Lipman, R.W. Baker and M.A. Johnson

Royal Free Hospital, London, UK

With a foreword by

P.A. Volberding

Professor and Vice-Chair of Medicine, UCSF
Chief, Medical Service, San Francisco Veterans
Affairs Medical Center
Co-Director, UCSF–GIVI Center for AIDS Research
San Francisco, CA, USA

The Parthenon Publishing Group

International Publishers in Medicine, Science & Technology

A CRC PRESS COMPANY

BOCA RATON   LONDON   NEW YORK   WASHINGTON, D.C.

Published in the USA by
The Parthenon Publishing Group
345 Park Avenue South, 10th Floor
New York
NY 10010
USA

Published in the UK and Europe by
The Parthenon Publishing Group
23–25 Blades Court
Deodar Road
London SW15 2NU
UK

Library of Congress Cataloging-in-Publication Data
Lipman, M. C. I.
    An atlas of differential diagnosis in HIV disease/M.C.I. Lipman, R. Baker and M.A.
    Johnson; with a foreword by P.A. Volberding.--2nd ed.
        p. ; cm -- (The Encyclopedia of visual medicine series)
    Includes bibliographical references and index.
    ISBN 1-84214-026-4 (alk, paper)
    1. AIDS (Disease)–Atlases. I. Title: Differential diagnosis in HIV disease. II. Baker, R.
    (Robert) III. Johnson, Margaret A., M.D. IV. Title. V. Series.
    [DNLM: 1. HIV Infections--diagnosis--Atlases. 2. Diagnosis, Differential--Atlases. WC
    17L766a2003]
    RC606.6.L.572003
    616.97'92075–dc22

                                                2003058104

British Library Cataloguing in Publication Data
Lipman, M. C. I.
    An atlas of differential diagnosis in HIV disease. - 2nd
    ed. - (The encyclopedia of visual medicine series)
    1.AIDS (Disease) - Diagnosis - Atlases 2.Diagnosis,
    Differential - Atlases
    I.Title II.Baker, R. III.Johnson, Margaret A.
    616.9'792'075

ISBN 1-84214-026-4

First published in 2004

Composition by The Parthenon Publishing Group
Printed and bound by T. G. Hostench S.A., Spain

Contents

Foreword

Much about the HIV/AIDS epidemic has not changed since publication of the first edition of *An Atlas of Differential Diagnosis in HIV Disease* in 1995. The virus is the same and, worldwide, most infected persons still progress to develop and die from the same range of opportunistic infections and malignancies. Yet, in other respects, it is a very different epidemic – in some respects almost unrecognizably so. For infected persons in wealthy economies, the use of prescribed multidrug antiretroviral regimens effectively blocks viral replication. In ideal cases such therapy prevents clinical progression durably, if not permanently. The most fortunate person with HIV infection might expect to begin therapy while still asymptomatic and avoid the immune deficiency and clinical problems of AIDS.

Many others infected with HIV – the vast majority worldwide – will have a very different experience. Their virus may already be drug resistant, allowing clinical progression despite therapy. Or, they might live in settings or circumstances where antiretroviral therapy is either unavailable, intermittently available, or not used. In fact, the dramatic explosion of the HIV epidemic in resource-limited settings will allow many more cases of clinical AIDS worldwide despite the advent of potent antiretroviral therapy. For these persons, the clinical conditions so well illustrated in *The Atlas of Differential Diagnosis in HIV Disease* will, sadly, remain as pertinent and important as ever.

But even the most fortunate HIV-infected person with full treatment access may still pose diagnostic challenges addressed in *The Atlas of Differential Diagnosis in HIV Disease*.

These patients are at risk for common, often striking, and potentially devastating complications representing drug toxicity or the consequences of prolonged survival with an incurable viral infection. These individuals may show striking fat atrophy or apparent fat accumulation. They may also have skin, hair, or nail changes or muscular atrophy from drug therapy.

The second edition of *The Atlas of Differential Diagnosis in HIV Disease* does an admirable job keeping abreast of such rapid and fundamental changes in the clinical presentation of HIV/AIDS. As with the previous edition, those opportunistic infections and malignancies are well covered. Excellent photographs and photomicrographs illustrate important clinical problems and the associated histological alterations. To keep pace with today's epidemic, however, crucial new information has been added. The worldwide HIV epidemiology, for example, is highlighted and another early section includes an excellent description – again, well illustrated – of the HIV life cycle and drug treatment targets.

Among the most significant additions to the current edition of *The Atlas of Differential Diagnosis in HIV Disease* are visually striking examples of the metabolic/morphological consequences of long-term HIV therapy. Cases include facial fat atrophy and central adiposity as well as computerized reconstructions of cosmetic therapy for these visual markers of HIV infection.

An Atlas of Differential Diagnosis in HIV Disease remains an important, accessible and striking work. It belongs in the library of each HIV expert and facility providing HIV care.

Paul A. Volberding, MD

Acknowledgements

Acknowledgements for first edition

We are grateful to our colleagues at the Royal Free Hospital, London, who kindly gave their time, expertise and permission to use material from their personal collections. In particular, we would like to thank:

Dr Alastair Deery, Department of Histopathology
Dr Bob Dick, Department of Radiology
Professor Allan MacLean, Department of Obstetrics and Gynaecology
Dr Jim McClaughlin, Department of Dermatology
Dr Alan Valentine, Department of Radiology
Dr Pauline Wilson, Department of Ophthalmology
Dr Tony Wilson, Department of Neurology

We are also indebted to the following for their help with this project:

Mr David Croser, Dental Surgeon, London
Dr Brian Gazzard and Dr Seng Lim, HIV/GUM Unit, Chelsea and Westminster Hospital, London
Dr Kitty Smith, The F.A.C.T.S Centre, London

The following also contributed material for which we are grateful:

Dr Roger Amos, Miss Clare Davey, Dr Owen Epstein, Dr Peggy Frith, Dr Gabriel Gabriel, Dr Stephen Gillespie, The Global AIDS Policy Coalition, Dr Mairhead Griffin, Dr Christine Lee, Dr David MacDonald-Burns, Dr Atul Mehta, Dr Deenan Pillay and Mr Mark Winslett.

We would also like to express our gratitude to all involved in HIV care at the Royal Free for their support of this work; especially Ms Greta Depledge for her formidable secretarial assistance. Thanks also to Nicola and Fiona for their tolerance.

We are indebted to Mr Richard Bowlby and the Department of Medical Illustration for their expert help in the preparation of the visual material.

This Atlas would never have been possible without those people with HIV and AIDS who kindly agreed to be photographed – and it is to our patients that we dedicate this book.

Acknowledgements for second edition

We wish to extend special thanks to our colleague Dr Pauline Wilson, Department of Ophthalmology, Royal Free Hospital who co-wrote the eye disease chapter.

Particular thanks are due also to the following who gave their time and expertise as well as images from their personal collections:

Dr Jamanda Haddock, Department of Radiology
Dr Mike Jarmulowicz, Department of Histopathology
Dr Jim McLaughlin, Department of Histopathology
Mr Juling Ong, Department of Plastic and Reconstructive Surgery
Dr Andy Platts, Department of Radiology

We are extremely grateful to the following who contributed material from their personal collections:

Professor Paul Griffiths, Department of Virology
Dr Sabine Kinloch, Department of Immunology
Dr Rob Miller, Patrick Manson Unit, University College London Hospitals
Dr Devi Nair, Department of Clinical Biochemistry

This project would never have reached fruition without the help and encouragement of our Editor, Pam Lancaster, as well as David Bloomer and all at Parthenon Publishing Group. For this we are most indebted.

I

HIV: an overview

No-one could have predicted the catastrophic course of the acquired immune deficiency syndrome (AIDS). Since the earliest reports of human immunodeficiency virus (HIV) in 1981 and the isolation of the pathogen in 1983, the scale of the crisis has confounded even the most pessimistic predictions. More than 20 million people have already died from HIV infection, and probably more than 60 million have been infected. Five million new infections occur every year, of which 800 000 are in children. This vulnerable group will often be left as orphans when their parents die of AIDS. However, they themselves account for 20% of all HIV-related deaths. In some sub-Saharan African countries, the median HIV prevalence among pregnant women in urban areas is in the order of 45%. About 70% of all new infections occur in sub-Saharan Africa, where the total number of people living with the disease exceeds 30 million. HIV/AIDS is the leading cause of death in Africa and the fourth biggest global killer (Figures 1.1 and 1.2).

While it is clear that the development and spread of the disease should be considered in decades rather than years, certain regions of the world may yet escape more lightly. In contrast to Southern Africa, Northern Africa and the Middle East still have a relatively low incidence and prevalence of HIV, as does Central Europe. However, the factors associated with rapid and explosive HIV spread – high levels of population mobility, political instability, risky sexual behavior – are present in many countries in these regions. This has already taken place in Eastern Europe, particularly Uzbekistan. It is becoming clear that HIV is far more common and widespread in the Republic of China than was officially acknowledged; the epidemics in South East Asia and Latin America

are well established. The predicted 'plateau' in prevalence in countries with uncontrolled epidemics has not yet materialized.

Until recently, the world has been almost completely unprepared for the economic and social impact of the epidemic. The loss of young and productive people within societies causes families, economies and eventually nations to falter and stumble. For countries with national HIV/AIDS prevalence rates of 20%, annual growth of GDP (gross domestic product) has been estimated to shrink by an average of 2.6 percentage points. The rate of economic growth has fallen by 2–4% in sub-Saharan Africa. Gains in longevity, painfully established since the 1950s through improved social conditions and public health programs, have been rapidly and tragically reversed in many developing nations.

The vast majority of HIV infections are spread through sexual contact. World-wide over 70% of infections are acquired heterosexually. In higher-income countries, homosexual/bisexual males account for the largest number of infected individuals, although the pattern is changing. In many western nations, transmission through heterosexual sex has overtaken transmission through sex between men as the principal route of new infections. In certain countries, notably Britain, this is at least in part due to immigrants and asylum-seekers from nations with a high prevalence of HIV. In some countries, sexual behavior would seem to be changing. In the USA, UK and Australia there is evidence of increased high-risk sexual behavior among both heterosexuals and men who have sex with men. In Japan, transmission of HIV through male–male sexual contact is increasing. Elsewhere,

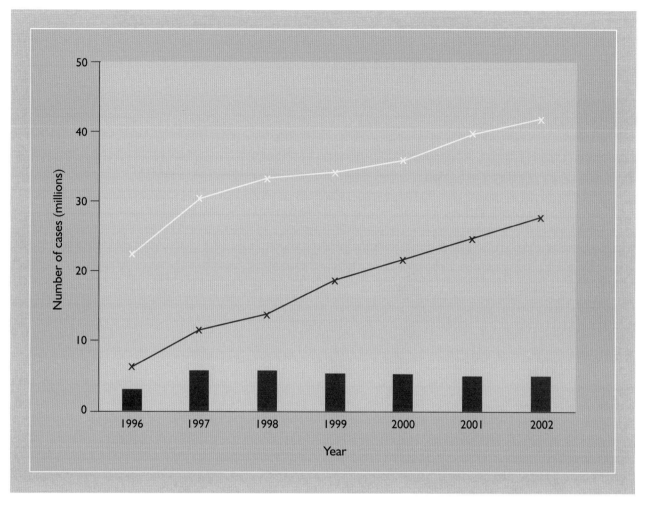

Figure 1.1 *Adult/pediatric HIV/AIDS cases* Estimated number of adults and children living with HIV/AIDS (orange); estimated cumulative number of deaths due to AIDS (purple); new HIV infections (red). Data from UNAIDS/WHO Joint United Nations Programme on HIV/AIDS

notably Spain, Portugal and Eastern Europe, transmission through contaminated needles among injecting drug users remains a major, preventable, route of infection.

Infectious virus can be recovered from blood, semen and cervical or vaginal secretions. For a given sexual episode, factors that increase the risk of acquiring HIV include the presence of genital ulceration and other sexually transmitted diseases, anal sex and traumatic vaginal sex. A European study that investigated heterosexual couples discordant for HIV estimated a risk per unprotected sex episode of 0.2% for male to female and 0.1% for female to male transmission. Similar work in Africa has suggested transmission rates to be between 10 and 100 times these figures. This may reflect increased infectivity (including increased

transmission from genital ulcer disease) or susceptibility factors, or differences in data collection. Within the homosexual community the introduction of 'safer sex' (i.e. sex involving either condom usage or low-risk activities) had led to a significant reduction in transmission of HIV infection. There is increasing evidence that this trend is reversing.

Injecting drug use is responsible for about 10% of all HIV infections; in some countries such as Portugal and Spain, the figure is higher. Injecting drug users are at increased risk of HIV infection if they share needles or take multiple drugs. Inadequately sterilized needles, re-used within a medical setting, can also lead to HIV infection. Less than 5% of all HIV infections result from infected blood and blood products. Within the developed world screening for

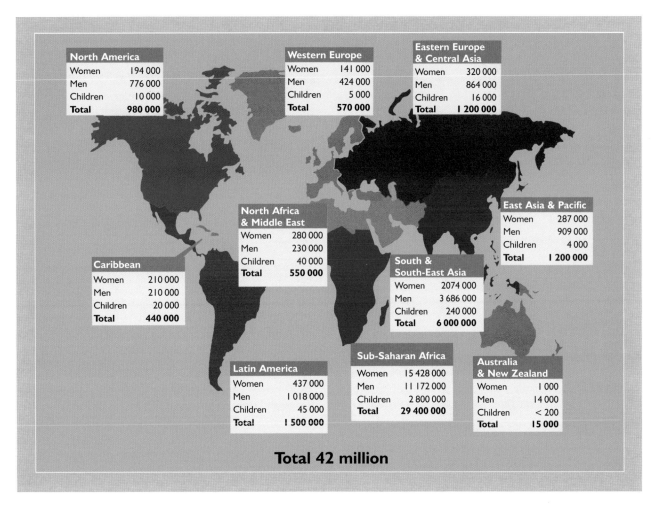

Figure 1.2   Adults and children estimated to be living with HIV/AIDS, end 2002. Data from UNAIDS/WHO. AIDS epidemic update, December 2002. Joint United Nations Programme on HIV/AIDS (UNAIDS) and World Health Organization (WHO). Geneva: UNAIDS, 2002

HIV has virtually eliminated the risk of acquiring HIV in this way. However, many developing countries still cannot afford to test their blood supply and some continue to pay individuals for blood donations. As a large number of paid donors come from high-risk groups, this practice has been associated with sustained infection within the blood supply.

Vertical HIV transmission can occur *in utero*, at the time of birth and during breastfeeding. The estimated rates of unprotected mother to child transmission vary from 15–25% in Europe to 25–40% in Africa. The risk of transmission may be increased by various specific factors (e.g. HIV strain or viral load), maternal factors (e.g. advanced stage of HIV infection or presence of sexually transmitted infections (STIs)) and local factors (e.g. mode of

delivery or breastfeeding). Conversely, risk reduction to less than 2% can occur with perinatal antiretroviral use, elective Cesarean section and avoidance of breastfeeding. On its own, the latter will halve rates of transmission, although, potentially, it also has a negative effect since the infant will not receive maternally derived passive immunity against other locally prevalent infections. In non-breastfeeding populations, approximately two-thirds of HIV transmission occurs at the time of birth.

Maternal HIV immunoglobulin G (IgG) antibody may be found in uninfected neonates and, therefore, neonatal antibody testing may be unreliable. However, 50% of HIV-negative children will have cleared this passively acquired antibody at 10 months and almost 100% by 18 months. By this time, however, 20% of infected children will have developed AIDS. Techniques which detect minute quantities of antigen such as polymerase chain reaction (PCR) may be positive as early as 3 months from birth in a child who is truly HIV-positive. Maternal–fetal HIV transmission is almost entirely preventable by comparatively simple strategies where there is the political will to implement them.

Within the developed world and, to a lesser extent, the developing nations, the advent of effective antiretroviral agents has transformed the evolution of the disease. Some 500 000 people are now believed to be taking highly active antiretroviral therapy (HAART) world-wide. Associated with this intervention, there has been a massive decrease in mortality: deaths in the USA fell by 42% in 1996–97, a year after its introduction, although the decline has now levelled off. HIV remains an incurable infection and the long-term prognosis for people taking suppressive medication remains a matter of speculation. However, clinicians in the higher-income nations report that the profile of morbidity encountered with HIV-infected patients has dramatically changed, and that gross, untreatable, opportunistic infections have become far less common.

The improvement in systemic immunity also means that many individuals who were taking infection prophylaxis can now stop this when their blood tests show sustained effects such as CD4 counts above $200 \times 10^6/l$ and low HIV load on repeat testing. The advantage for the individual of reducing pill burden and minimizing side-effects and potential drug interactions are immense.

The unforeseen consequence of HAART has been greater numbers of surviving individuals with high morbidity from chronic infections such as hepatitis B and C. The complexities of co-infection require skilled medical care. There are also significant numbers of individuals suffering both short- and long-term toxicity from antiretroviral medication.

The use of drug therapy has led to antiretroviral resistance. This has proven to be an economic and intellectual demand on health-care providers. New techniques of analyzing genotypic and phenotypic viral resistance have had to be developed. These have added to our understanding of HIV infection. However, the large-scale production of HAART in fewer tablets with less dietary and storage restrictions is also important, as this improves adherence to medication – a major factor in determining the development of resistance. Efforts to reduce the cost of HAART to make it a realistic proposition in resource-poor settings have met with limited success. It remains to be seen what will be the consequences of providing HAART without the technical facilities to monitor host and viral responses.

Despite the apparent catastrophic spread of what is an eminently preventable infection, there is some cause for hope world-wide. Thailand has shown that intervention can modify the evolution of the epidemic; the number of new infections was reduced from 143 000 in 1991 to 29 000 in 2001. Certain Central European countries, notably Poland, have prevented the epidemic from spreading into the wider population by successfully controlling it among injecting drug users. Public awareness programs in Uganda, Zambia and Côte d'Ivoire are showing some evidence of bearing fruit. The position of the Government of South Africa in denying that HIV is the cause of AIDS has held back useful and life-saving interventions from its people.

Controlling the epidemic is, of course, largely a question of prevention. Addressing the many political, social, cultural and economic factors that render populations and individuals susceptible to the disease is central to the international response. However, treatment of infected individuals is a basic necessity. Even in settings where antiretrovirals are not a realistic option, the management of opportunistic infections, notably tuberculosis, can significantly improve morbidity and mortality.

The Declaration of Commitment on HIV/AIDS was adopted by the world's governments at the Special Session of the United Nations General Assembly on HIV/AIDS in June 2001. It established, for the first time ever, time-bound targets to which governments and the United Nations may be held accountable. An example of this is a reduction in the incidence of childhood HIV infections by 20% and 50% in 2005 and 2010, respectively. There is at last evidence that the world is making some effort to come to terms with the disaster that has befallen it.

SUBTYPES OF HIV

Two subtypes (HIV-1 and HIV-2) have been identified. HIV-1 is responsible for the vast majority of infections, while HIV-2 is mainly prevalent in West Africa and appears to have a similar but rather slower clinical course. This Atlas deals predominantly with HIV-1 infection.

The virus shows remarkable genetic and molecular adaptability. In order to map its genetic variation of HIV-1, the virus has been classified by molecular biologists into three groups: M (main), O (outlier) and N (non-M, non-O).

The M group is further classified into a number of subtypes, defined as having genomes that are at least 25% unique. These are designated by a letter, A, B, C, for example, and so far, 11 have been identified. There are also variants resulting from the blending which may arise when an individual is infected with two different HIV subtypes. These are known as 'circulating recombinant forms' (CRF). To date, 13 have been identified. The subtypes and CRFs provide useful means of tracking the route of the epidemic. All subtypes as well as some CRFs occur in Africa. In Europe, America and Australia, subtype B is most common, with subtype C being more common in Africa and India. Subtypes C and A are most common overall.

There is continuing debate over whether certain subtypes are more or less aggressive or transmissible. It is also not clear whether differences in response to antiretrovirals occur between subtypes. Most data until now have predictably been limited to treatment of subtype B, because it is the most common in wealthier countries.

HIV also constantly mutates at a very high rate within individuals. There is constant background mutation and variation. This will be affected by external pressures, such as the individual immune response or exposure to antiretroviral drugs. Mutation has important consequences in terms both of developing resistance to antiretroviral agents and of vaccine production. Both of these are discussed elsewhere.

PREVENTION STRATEGIES

Controlling the spread of HIV requires a concerted effort at both a global and local level. The most important measures are:

(1) Promotion of the use of condoms in all sexually active people (regardless of HIV status);

(2) Provision of needle and syringe exchanges and safer sex information for injecting drug users;

(3) Provision of appropriate contraceptive advice for seropositive women, if possible, using assisted means of conception to reduce the risk of fetal infection;

(4) Provision of HIV screening for all pregnant women or, ideally, women considering conception;

(5) Provision of appropriate advice on delivery technique and avoidance of breastfeeding for seropositive women;

(6) Provision of appropriate antiretroviral medication for seropositive pregnant women prior to parturition and antiretrovirals for neonates in some cases;

(7) Provision of a safe supply of blood and blood products;

(8) Treatment of other sexually transmitted diseases;

(9) Provision of sex education in schools and the community in an understandable form, including the removal of stigma from HIV infection;

(10) Mobilization of communities to develop partnerships between social and governmental organizations which systematically involve individuals infected by or affected by HIV/AIDS;

(11) Addressing, at national and international levels, the economic, political, social and cultural factors that render individuals and communities vulnerable to HIV/AIDS.

The fear that sex education and distribution of condoms or needles to high-risk groups would increase risk behavior is unfounded. These social programs justify their cost by reducing the need for expensive HIV treatment, and by reducing the economic burden that widespread HIV infection exacts from the community.

RISK TO HEALTH-CARE WORKERS

HIV is much less infectious than either hepatitis B or C. Casual contact (e.g. physical examination) carries no risk of infection; the rate of transmission by parenteral exposure is approximately 3 per 1000 cases (0.3%). The risk from exposure to mucous membrane or non-intact skin is too low to be currently quantified. The majority of documented HIV seroconversions in health-care workers have occurred in nurses and laboratory technicians via percutaneous hollow-bore needlestick injury. None of these were superficial scratches and the majority

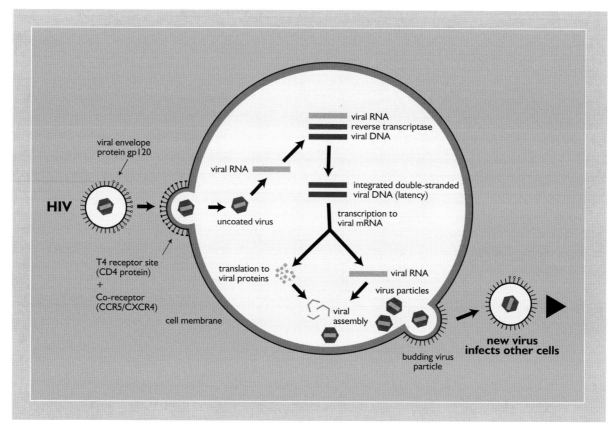

Figure 1.3   Schematic representation of HIV replication

were deep wounds. The risk of nosocomial HIV transmission can be reduced by adopting 'universal precautions', including double-gloving and protective eye wear. Disposal of needles should be carried out immediately and without resheathing. Regular 'safety at work' courses are important for all staff. The risk of transmission of HIV from an infected health-care worker to a patient approaches zero, despite numerous large, expensive 'lookback' studies in many countries.

VIROLOGY AND IMMUNOLOGY OF HIV

HIV is a human retrovirus belonging to the lentivirus family. Binding of the HIV-1 external envelope glycoprotein gp120 to the CD4 receptor on human cells is the first step in HIV–cell interaction and virus entry (Figure 1.3). Cell-free or cell-associated HIV infects cells through attachment of the viral envelope proteins (gp120 and gp41) to the CD4 antigen complex on host cells. HIV gp120 must bind to a cell surface protein co-receptor called chemokine receptor 5 (CCR5) or other co-receptors, including CXCR4 and possibly CCR2, depending on host cell type. Polymorphisms within genes for CCR5 may affect disease progression by reducing the ability of HIV to enter and infect cells. The CD4 receptor is found on many cells, including T helper lymphocytes ('CD4 cells'), B lymphocytes, monocytes and tissue macrophages. Once HIV is inside the cell, it can, using viral reverse transcriptase, integrate its genetic material into the host genome. The virus (in the form of proviral DNA) remains latent in many cells until the cell itself becomes activated. This may arise from cytokine or antigen stimulation (e.g. with HIV or other viruses). The viral genetic material is then transcribed into new RNA which ultimately produces more infectious virus particles. These can leave the cell and infect other CD4-bearing cells.

How HIV infection leads to progressive immune dysfunction and AIDS is the subject of continuing debate. At initial infection, HIV spreads to the lymph nodes, circulating immune cells and thymus.

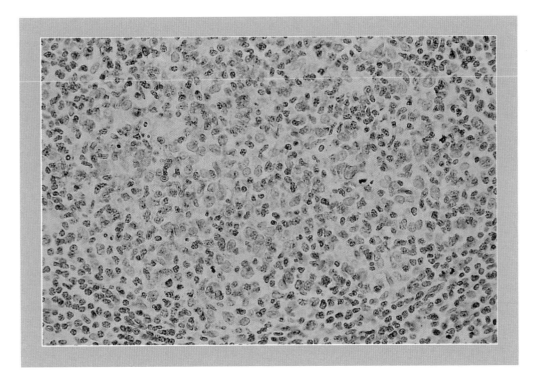

Figure 1.4   Follicular dendritic cells staining yellow from HIV antigen surface deposition in a lymph node biopsy

The acute viremia is partly cleared by a strong host immune response (involving both cell-mediated and humoral mechanisms). Within the germinal centers of the lymph nodes, the follicular dendritic cells (FDC) attempt to trap HIV on their cell surface, resulting in follicular hyperplasia and expansion of the FDC network. Figure 1.4 shows FDCs staining yellow from HIV antigen surface deposition in a lymph node biopsy.

At this stage, the patient is clinically well although there is usually detectable virus in the blood. With time, persistent infection in the lymph node produces progressive degeneration of the FDC network and plasma HIV load may increase. The immune system has become damaged by HIV, and is unable to control the widespread dissemination and replication of the virus. This is mirrored by CD4 cell depletion and the onset of clinical symptoms. The immune dysregulation ultimately results in opportunistic infections and tumors.

The host immune responses produced against HIV do not appear to be adequate to control the virus. This may reflect its persistence within cells such as monocytes/macrophages acting as 'reservoirs of HIV'. Furthermore, because HIV 'targets' the immune system the host response is abnormal. Examples of this include a reduction in number and functional capacity of circulating T helper cells, impaired or abnormal cytotoxic T-cell responses and a persisting polyclonal hypergammaglobulinemia.

Perinatally infected children are somewhat different to adults as here HIV infection occurs before the immune system has fully developed. The infecting strain is one that has evaded maternal immune responses and is, therefore, less likely to promote useful host reactions in the child. A reflection of this is the failure to control acute HIV viremia during perinatal seroconversion.

A number of theories have been developed to explain how HIV infection results in the destruction or loss of peripheral CD4 cells.

Syncytia formation

In vitro, a few HIV-infected CD4 cells can fuse with uninfected CD4 cells, forming a syncytium. This leads to the death of all the cells. It is not known whether syncytium formation is actually important *in vivo*.

Production of gp120

While HIV is replicating in CD4 cells, there is excessive production of the HIV cell surface glycoprotein gp120. This could attach to CD4 molecules on uninfected cells and may render them susceptible to antibody-mediated or cytotoxic attack. CD4 cells that have gp120 bound to them may be functionally abnormal.

Apoptosis

HIV-infected CD4 cells seem to be excessively programmed for apoptosis. The reason is unclear but one possibility is that HIV antigens act as superantigens, causing non-specific polyclonal activation of large numbers of CD4 cells. The cytokine milieu will affect the rate of apoptosis, with interleukin-1 (IL-1) and tumor necrosis factor (TNF) promoting cell death and IL-2 being protective.

Recent research has suggested that apoptosis of infected, resting T cells follows programming which directs the cells 'home' to the lymph nodes. Subsequently, HIV can leave permanent fibrosis within lymph nodes and destroy the T-cell zone, which is vital to the production of new CD4 cells.

MHC and gp120 homology: autoimmunity

There is functional homology between subunits of gp120 and host major histocompatibility complex (MHC) molecules. Where there is free gp120 circulating it may bind to CD4 cells, mimicking the action of MHC when a further antigen is encountered. This may explain excessive T-cell activation in HIV and this may be associated with increased replication of HIV as well.

A further controversial but related theory for CD4 destruction involves the failure of recognition of CD4 cells as 'self' and induction of cytotoxic autoimmunity. HIV antigens may, in this context, mimic the activity of foreign MHC molecules. Once again, this could explain excessive and unsuppressed immunological activation during HIV infection. Thrombocytopenia, arthritis, psoriasis, vasculitis and dermatitis all occur in HIV infection and may well be autoimmune in etiology.

Chronic immune activation

Replication of HIV drives the proliferation of both CD4 and CD8 cells within the lymphoreticular system. This leads to trapping of T cells within lymph nodes and may explain why there is an apparent increase in total body T cells but a fall in blood CD4 cells. Control of HIV leads to a decrease in T-cell activation, the markers of which can accurately predict individual response to therapy independent of plasma viral load (e.g. CD8, CD38).

Graft-versus-host disease

There are similarities between infection with HIV and the syndrome which occurs when foreign, transplanted tissue attacks the transplant host. Dermatitis, diarrhea, enlarged lymph nodes and a risk of developing lymphomas are common to both HIV infection and graft-versus-host disease. Changes in cytokine profiles are similar in both.

TESTING FOR HIV

Discussion of pre- and post-test HIV should provide individuals with information about the HIV test as well as the implications of the result. It also gives an opportunity to educate people about methods of transmission and discuss behavior that may reduce their risks. The particular context of the test may determine the time and detail of the discussion, although informed consent is mandatory. If an individual tests HIV antibody-positive, then a counselling/clinical psychology service can provide important non-medical support, both acutely and in the longer term.

HIV antibody tests

Almost everybody forms antibodies to HIV within 6 months of infection, and in the majority of infections, this happens by 6 weeks. Up to 70% will have a seroconversion illness. HIV IgG antibody will normally be detectable within 2–3 weeks of the occurrence of the symptoms. An IgM response occurs earlier, but is not always present. A very small number of people may take longer than 6 months to produce antibodies and, if there is clinical suspicion of HIV, repeat antibody testing is required until 1 year after the last exposure.

There are now many different means of testing for HIV, each with its own advantages and disadvantages. Strategies for HIV antibody testing should aim for maximum accuracy but minimum cost. The principal tests in common use are given below.

ELISA

The presence of HIV antibodies is established by a color change in a microtiter plate. This reflects the presence or absence of antibodies bound to an enzyme which alters the color of an indicator solution. This was the first commonly used test for antibodies and is relatively easy to perform. It is time-consuming and is not well designed for one-off, rapid testing. Commercial tests typically include a range of antigens to cover HIV-1 (group M) and HIV-2 and, increasingly, HIV-1 group O as well.

Competitive ELISA

HIV antibodies, if present, have to compete with known antibodies added to the test well. High concentrations of HIV antibody in the tested serum will prevent the other antibodies, which are bound to the indicator-changing enzyme, from binding. Thus, no color change represents a positive test.

Third- and fourth-generation assays (sandwich tests)

These rely on multiple binding sites in HIV antibodies, one site binding to the test antigen and another to a labelled antigen. They have the advantage of being fast, easy to automate and sensitive to low concentrations of antibody, including IgM present in early infection. The test may be combined with p24 antigen ('Gag' protein) assay.

Western blot (Figure 1.5)

Once believed to be the most reliable of tests for HIV, it is now clear that this test – as well as being expensive, subjective in interpretation and time-consuming – does generate false-positive results. It involves placing multiple enzyme-bound antigens on a nitrocellulose plate; the antigen bands change color when bound to specific HIV antibody. It has the advantage of simultaneously testing for multiple HIV antibodies. However, there may be cross-reactivity with autoimmune diseases, recent vaccinations and so-called endogenous retroviruses. P24 antigen may also cross-react with

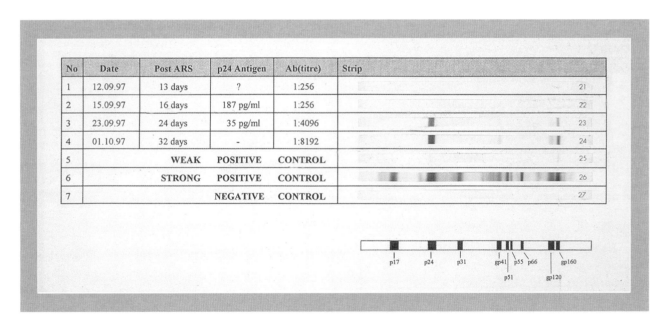

No	Date	Post ARS	p24 Antigen	Ab(titre)	Strip
1	12.09.97	13 days	?	1:256	21
2	15.09.97	16 days	187 pg/ml	1:256	22
3	23.09.97	24 days	35 pg/ml	1:4096	23
4	01.10.97	32 days	-	1:8192	24
5		WEAK	POSITIVE	CONTROL	25
6		STRONG	POSITIVE	CONTROL	26
7			NEGATIVE	CONTROL	27

Figure 1.5 Sequential Western blots in an individual with primary HIV infection. The image shows four serial blood samples obtained from a patient 13–32 days after the onset of a flu-like illness (acute retroviral syndrome, ARS). Whilst with time there is variable detection of p24 antigen by ELISA, the Western blot strip reveals increasing amounts of p24, gp120 and gp160, indicating HIV antibody positivity. HIV-positive and -negative controls are run concurrently – shown in rows 5, 6 and 7

cytomegalovirus (CMV) within this system. Western blot is therefore best used as one confirmatory strand in a testing strategy.

Immunofluorescence

Previously HIV-infected cells (and uninfected controls) are exposed to test serum. Antibodies will only bind to infected cells; subsequently, further antibodies bound to fluorescent stains are added. The cell–antibody–stain complexes glow. This is a very quick but subjective test.

Urine and saliva tests

These are used principally for research as they are more expensive and less reliable than blood testing.

Sensitivity and specificity

The World Health Organization (WHO) has issued guidelines on sensitivity and specificity of antibody testing for HIV. For screening purposes, ELISA kits should not be used unless they can detect 100% of known positive samples in a reference panel of 203 HIV-1 and/or 60 HIV-2 samples.

Where the aim is to establish quickly the HIV status of an individual, rather than screening, say, blood products, 99% sensitivity is considered to be adequate.

WHO does not recommend the use of tests with a specificity of less than 95%. African serum of known positivity is used as a reference range. Most kits exceed this standard, but the possibility of false-positives means that a second test must always be performed using different antigens. A competitive ELISA or another kit using different antigens or immunofluorescence/Western blotting may be used.

HIV antigen tests

There are a number of reasons for wanting to identify, quantify or culture viral antigen. As stated, it may be necessary to look for viral antigen in exposed persons during the 'window' period, before an antibody response develops. HIV viral load is measured as a means of monitoring response to antiretroviral medication and defining an individual's risk of progression. When treatment fails, it may be necessary to examine the genome or the phenotype of the virus to identify resistant strains.

Molecular techniques, such as PCR, amplify RNA from virions in plasma. There are, at present, two main assays: the Roche PCR assay and the Chiron/Bayer bDNA assay. Each test has particular characteristics, and results from different test kits may not be strictly comparable.

Amplicor® HIV-1 Monitor

The Roche PCR test is called the Amplicor HIV-1 Monitor (Roche Molecular Systems, Inc., Pleasanton, CA, USA). The standard Amplicor assay has a lower detection limit of 400 RNA copies/ml, whereas the ultrasensitive assay can detect virus above 50 copies/ml. The Amplicor assay detects subtypes B, C and D.

Quantiplex®/Versant® 3.0 bDNA assay

The branched-chain DNA (or bDNA for short) test, marketed under the tradename Quantiplex 3.0 (Bayer plc, Strawberry Hill, Berkshire, UK) in Europe or Versant 3.0 (Bayer Diagnostics, Tarrytown, NY, USA) in the USA, has a lower detection limit of 50 bDNA copies and an upper limit of 500 000 bDNA. The standard version of this test is the Quantiplex 2.0 bDNA assay which has a lower limit of detection of 500 copies/ml. The ultrasensitive Quantiplex 3.0 assay may be more sensitive than the Amplicor ultrasensitive test for measuring low levels of HIV; there may also be less variability using the Quantiplex system.

Ultrasensitive tests

Viral suppression below the ultrasensitive detection range of 50 copies/ml is associated with sustained long-term viral suppression. Many individuals with viral loads below 400 are subsequently found to have detectable virus with more sensitive tests. Ultrasensitive viral load tests are more useful in assessing the effects of treatment than standard assays. Future tests will detect less than 10 copies/ml. The advantage of these assays remains to be determined.

Molecular techniques are also used for detecting mutations associated with resistance; this is discussed below.

Viral cultures

HIV from both plasma and infected cells can be cultured in donor cells. It is a time-consuming technique principally used for research.

Resistance testing

Assays for testing for drug resistance in HIV-1 infection are now available and clinical studies suggest that viral drug resistance is correlated both with failure of current therapy and with poor virologic response to new therapy. Because of assay complexities and expense, it is likely that testing will remain centralized in large commercial laboratories.

Genotypic tests

Many mutation patterns associated with resistance to specific drugs have been identified. Genotype testing detects mutations that confer phenotypic resistance. These can be assessed using a number of techniques. The assays depend upon amplification of HIV-1 sequences from plasma containing at least 500–1000 HIV RNA copies/ml. Genotypic assays may differentiate a mutant at a level of 10–50% in a mixture of viruses. The commonly used techniques are molecular assays, which use specific primers to amplify known mutations, point mutation assays and line probe assays, which amplify codons. Both of these latter techniques suffer from the disadvantage that the resistance mutations need to be known in advance. Genotypic sequences may also be established by automated gene sequencers.

There are a number of drawbacks to genotypic resistance testing techniques in practice (Figure 1.6). They require experience and skill to interpret. They are not fully validated and there is variability between laboratories. However, recent reports have shown high concordance for genotype results between two experienced laboratories. Resistance tests may be unreliable at lower viral loads of less than 1000 copies/ml, and where antiretrovirals have been stopped. Continuing antiretroviral therapy provides selection pressure for resistant mutants, which may not reproduce effectively when that pressure is removed. The resistant virus may recur when the challenge is reintroduced.

Phenotypic tests

These tests measure the ability of plasma viral HIV-1 isolate to grow in the presence of drugs. The degree of inhibition of viral replication at different drug concentrations is assessed. Results are used to calculate the 50% or 90% inhibitory concentration (IC50 or IC90) of a drug for an isolate. The recombinant virus IC50 for each drug is expressed relative to

specific reference wild HIV strains (NL4-3 or HXB-2). An increase in IC50 of more than four-fold that of the reference strain is reported as reduced susceptibility. Such tests are now feasible via rapid, high-throughput automated assays based on recombinant DNA technology. RNA can be amplified and multiple drugs may be tested simultaneously.

These assays only amplify the most common circulating viral clones (Figure 1.7). Less predominant drug-resistant species (< 10–50% of the viral population), which could contribute to drug failure or transmission of resistant HIV, may not be detected.

INVESTIGATION AND FOLLOW-UP OF A NEW HIV-SEROPOSITIVE INDIVIDUAL

Baseline investigations are summarized in Figure 1.8. The important aspects of medical care in a confirmed HIV-positive patient include:

(1) Determination of the stage of their disease through history, examination and laboratory tests;

(2) Education about risk reduction, lifestyle management and the role of therapeutic interventions, about HIV itself and the importance of adherence in drug treatment;

(3) Consideration of the issues that are of importance to specific groups (e.g. cervical smears in women, rehabilitation programs in injecting drug users).

People with HIV infection should have easy access to medical care. The frequency of medical review depends on their stage of disease, and whether they are taking HAART. Typically, an asymptomatic HIV-positive person may be seen 3–6-monthly. At this time, clinical assessment and laboratory monitoring should be performed (e.g. immune markers, viral load, hematological and biochemical screens). Patients initiating antiretroviral therapy for the first time, or with adherence difficulties, should be seen more frequently.

NATURAL HISTORY OF HIV INFECTION

The advent of HAART in 1995/96 altered the progress of HIV infection for many individuals.

Advantages	Disadvantages
Less complex test	May be less useful for resistance to protease inhibitors
Less expensive	May need expert interpretation
More widely available	Most cannot detect minor species
Works at a lower viral load	Links between genes and resistance not fully understood
More rapid results	Laboratory quality varies
	Must be on anti-HIV therapy

Figure 1.6   Advantages and disadvantages of genotypic resistance testing

Advantages	Disadvantages
Directly measures drug effect	Complex test
Easier to interpret	Cannot detect minor species
Information on cross-resistance	Must be on HIV therapy

Figure 1.7   Advantages and disadvantages of phenotypic resistance testing

Mortality from HIV plummeted within the space of little more than a single year. Death rates within the large EuroSida cohort fell from 23.3 deaths to 4.1 per 100 person-years between September 1994 and March 1998. There is no doubt that HAART is a cost-effective and worthwhile intervention. However, a brief review of the epidemiology and economics of HIV indicates that the use of HAART remains largely confined to the wealthier nations. For the vast majority of infected people, the natural history of HIV is much the same as in the pre-HAART era.

Without antiretrovirals in the developed world, the median interval between HIV seroconversion and progression to AIDS in adults is estimated to be 10 years, with a range of between 18 months and 25 years. It is now believed that almost all individuals would, eventually, develop AIDS if left untreated. However, there is great variation between individuals and groups in this respect. Untreated, 94% of AIDS patients would die within 5 years, even

with access to western health care. Approximately 20% of perinatally infected children in richer nations will develop rapidly progressive symptomatic disease (usually *Pneumocystis* pneumonia) or show developmental delay or regression in their first year of life. The other four-fifths have an untreated median survival of 9 years. In Africa, it is estimated that up to 80% of children will be dead within three years of infection.

The fall in blood absolute CD4 T lymphocyte count is the most widely used prognostic marker. However, these are affected by a number of factors apart from HIV (e.g. intercurrent infection, smoking, exercise, time of day and laboratory variation). CD4 percentage is a more stable measure, and can be used if CD4 absolute counts appear to vary widely from visit to visit. The rate of decline of CD4 cells is a better marker and combining this with absolute CD4 counts yields more information. It should be remembered that CD4 counts are significantly

Investigation	Reason for investigation
Virology	
Confirmatory HIV antibody	confirmation
HIV viral load	prognostic marker
CMV antibody	? cofactor; previous exposure; risk of future disease
Hepatitis screen (A, B and C)	may develop chronic disease; hepatitis A and B vaccination may be required
CMV viral load	risk of end-organ disease, CD4 < 100 x 10^6/l
Immunology	
T-lymphocyte subsets	prognostic marker
Microbiology	
Syphilis serology (EIA/RPR/TPHA/FTA)	occult/latent disease
Toxoplasma serology (dye test)	previous exposure; risk of future disease
Biochemistry	
Urea, electrolytes and creatinine	baseline
Liver function tests	abnormal with disease or drug therapy
Glucose, amylase, thyroid function tests	baseline
Lipid profile	baseline; lipid-altering drugs may be prescribed
Hematology	
Full blood count	HIV-related hematological abnormalities/drug therapy
Differential film	
Cytology	
Cervical smear	higher incidence of cervical cancer
Chest radiograph	occult disease; baseline
Dental check-up	higher incidence of dental disease

EIA, enzyme immunoassay; RPR, rapid plasma reagin; TPHA, *Treponema pallidum* hemagglutination test; FTA, fluorescent treponemal antibody test

Figure 1.8   Baseline investigations of a new HIV-seropositive individual

higher in infants and that CD4-based 'risk stratification' needs to be adjusted for the child's age.

It is now well established that high viral loads are associated with more rapid disease progression and risk of death. The pathogenicity of the virus itself may also indicate the risk of opportunistic disease. For example, patients from whom syncytium-inducing (SI) viral strains can be grown in cell culture have a six times increased risk of progression to AIDS compared with those with non-SI strains over a 30-month period. Reports that certain HIV subtypes may be associated with a more aggressive disease course, or that the virus may be mutating to become more aggressive, have not been confirmed. However, viral recombinations and superinfection with subsequent rapid progression have been documented.

HIV-related clinical symptoms provide important prognostic information independent of CD4 count. Most studies have shown that oral thrush and constitutional symptoms (e.g. malaise, idiopathic fever, night sweats, diarrhea and weight loss) are the strongest clinical predictors of progression to AIDS. These features were previously described as part of the AIDS-related complex (ARC).

For a given adult, of all the demographic and lifestyle factors examined, only age (> 35 years at time of seroconversion) and baseline albumin levels (< 35 mg/l) appear clearly to worsen the outcome.

Descriptive classification systems are widely used for disease reporting, although, unlike staging systems, they cannot predict individual outcomes. The US Centers for Disease Control and Prevention (CDC) clinical classification of disease is the best known and is based on evidence of HIV infection with clinical indicators of impairment in cell-mediated immunity (Figure 1.9).

AIDS itself is a surveillance definition and has therefore been modified to incorporate the expanding spectrum of recognized opportunist disease (Figure 1.10).

The 1993 CDC classification included an immunological criterion for AIDS (CD4 count < 200 x 10^6/l or CD4 percentage < 14%) irrespective of clinical symptoms (Figure 1.11).

Long-term follow-up studies suggested that a proportion of patients will remain asymptomatic (approximately 20% at 10 years). However, very few of these people have stable CD4 counts. Furthermore, patients will often have minor symptoms and signs suggesting immune dysfunction.

Examples of these include new or worsening skin rashes (including herpes), tiredness, cough and low-grade anemia. In the majority of infected people, the absolute CD4 count falls with time. Figure 1.12 shows a 'schematic' CD4 count decline and the points below which common opportunist diseases may be expected to occur.

It is important to consider HIV infection in an individual of unknown status who presents with any of these conditions. This also applies to children with lymphadenopathy or hepatosplenomegaly of unknown cause, persistent parotid swelling, skin disease such as shingles or extensive molluscum contagiosum, thrombocytopenia, recurrent infections or failure to thrive.

Apart from sex-related conditions such as cervical carcinoma, AIDS indicator diseases generally do not appear to differ between men and women. However, some conditions are much more common in certain risk groups. Injecting drug users have a high incidence of wasting syndrome, recurrent bacterial pneumonia and tuberculosis. Geographic differences in diseases occur, which reflect the opportunistic pathogens present in the local environment (e.g. histoplasmosis or visceral leishmaniasis usually only occur in individuals from endemic areas). In the developed world, gender, racial and HIV risk factor survival differences after an AIDS diagnosis are determined by the degree of access to medical care. Studies have also shown that the level of experience of the doctor supervising treatment will also affect outcome.

Long-term non-progressors (defined as having HIV infection for more than 7 years with no history of HIV-related symptoms, normal blood CD4 count and no use of HAART) are relatively rare (less than 10% of most study populations). There is evidence that the route of infection can affect disease progress – people who acquire HIV by blood transfusion may have a worse outcome. Mutations in viral proteins such as Vpr are associated with less pathogenic strains, and perhaps a better prognosis. HIV in the developing world seems to pursue a more rapid course; this may be related to other cofactors, both infectious and non-infectious. Genetic factors are clearly important – the CCR5 co-receptor Δ32 mutation is associated with a reduced risk of progression to AIDS. There are also HLA associations which appear to influence disease progression.

Group I	acute primary infection
Group II	asymptomatic infection
Group III	persistent generalized lymphadenopathy (PGL)
Group IV	other disease
subgroup A	constitutional disease
	weight loss > 10% body weight or > 4.5 kg
	fevers > 38°C
	diarrhea lasting > 1 month
subgroup B	neurological disease
	myelopathy
	peripheral neuropathy
	HIV encephalopathy
subgroup C	secondary infectious diseases
	C1 AIDS-defining secondary infectious disease, e.g.
	Pneumocystis jiroveci pneumonia
	cerebral toxoplasmosis
	cytomegalovirus retinitis
	C2 other specified secondary infectious diseases, e.g.
	oral *Candida*
	multidermatomal varicella zoster
subgroup D	secondary cancers
	Kaposi's sarcoma
	non-Hodgkin's lymphoma
subgroup E	other conditions
	lymphoid interstitial pneumonitis

Figure 1.9   Centers for Disease Control classification of HIV infection (1985)

N.B. The CDC definition of the stages of HIV disease was updated in 1993. However, the older classification remains in use for some research studies and is therefore reproduced here

In those countries where HAART is available, the spectrum of HIV-related disease has changed. In the EuroSida cohort, opportunistic infections associated with very low CD4 counts – CMV retinitis and *Mycobacterium avium complex* (MAC), for example, are far less common. Malignant disease such as non-Hodgkin's lymphoma has increased as a proportion of all cases from 4% of all AIDS-defining events in 1994 to 16% in 1998.

Although death rates have fallen in HAART-treated populations, there has been an increase in the proportion of non-AIDS deaths. In some series, this accounts for the majority of events. The causes include liver disease and cancers, as well as

Clinical categories

Category A one or more of the conditions listed below in an adolescent or adult (13 years or older) with documented HIV infection. Conditions listed in Categories B and C must not have occurred.

Asymptomatic HIV infection

Persistent generalized lymphadenopathy (PGL)

Acute (primary) HIV infection with accompanying illness (sometimes known as seroconversion illness) or history of acute HIV infection

Category B symptomatic conditions in an HIV-infected adolescent or adult that are not included among conditions listed in Category C and that meet one of the following criteria:

a) The conditions are attributed to HIV infection or are indicative of a defect in cell-mediated immunity, or b) the conditions are considered by physicians to have a clinical course or to require management that is complicated by HIV infection. This category includes all such symptomatic conditions, with the exception of those placed in Category C.

Examples of conditions in this category include, but are not limited to:

Bacillary angiomatosis

Candidiasis (thrush) in the mouth and/or upper throat

Candidiasis of the vagina and/or vulva which is persistent, frequent, or responds poorly to treatment

Cervical abnormalities of moderate or severe extent or cervical cancer

Constitutional symptoms such as fever (38.5 °C) or diarrhea lasting longer than 1 month

Herpes zoster (shingles) involving at least two distinct episodes or more than one dermatome (skin area)

Idiopathic thrombocytopenia purpura

Listeriosis

Oral hairy leukoplakia

Pelvic inflammatory disease, particularly if complicated by tubo-ovarian abscess

Peripheral neuropathy

For classification purposes, Category B conditions take precedence over those in Category A. For example, someone previously treated for oral or persistent vaginal candidiasis (and who has not developed a Category C disease) but who is now asymptomatic should be classified in clinical Category B.

Category C includes the following conditions listed in the AIDS surveillance case definition. For classification purposes, once a Category C condition has occurred, the person will remain in Category C.

Candida in the esophagus, trachea, bronchi or lungs

Invasive cervical cancer

Coccidiodomycosis

Cryptococcus outside the lungs

Cryptosporidiosis with diarrhea lasting for more than 1 month

Cytomegalovirus disease outside the liver, spleen or lymph nodes

Cytomegalovirus retinitis

Herpes simplex virus causing prolonged skin problems or involving the lungs or esophagus

HIV-related encephalopathy

Chronic intestinal isosporiasis lasting longer than 1 month

Kaposi's sarcoma

Burkitt's, immunoblastic or primary (i.e. not involving other parts of the body) brain lymphoma

Widespread *Mycobacterium avium intracellulare* (MAC), *M. kansasii* or other species

Pneumocystis jiroveci pneumonia (PCP)

Recurrent bacterial pneumonia

Progressive multifocal leukoencephalopathy (PML)

Recurrent salmonella septicemia

Toxoplasmosis of the brain

HIV wasting syndrome

Figure 1.10   Centers for Disease Control clinical classification of disease (1993) with AIDS indicator diseases (Category C)

	Clinical category		
	A	*B*	*C*
CD4 T-cell categories	*Acute (primary) HIV, asymptomatic or PGL*	*Symptomatic (not A or C – see explanation)*	*AIDS indicator conditions*
≥ 500 x 10⁶/l	A1	B1	C1
200–499 x 10⁶/l	A2	B2	C2
< 200 x 10⁶/l	A3	B3	C3

PGL, persistent generalized lymphadenopathy

This classification stratifies patients clinically (A–C) and immunologically (1–3). Groups A3 and B3 satisfy the immunological but not the clinical criteria for AIDS. Category B consists of symptomatic conditions that are not included in category C but can be either attributed to, or are complicated by, HIV infection. Examples include thrush (oral or persistent vulvovaginal), moderate or severe cervical dysplasia, thrombocytopenia and peripheral neuropathy

Figure 1.11   1993 Revised CDC classification system for HIV infection

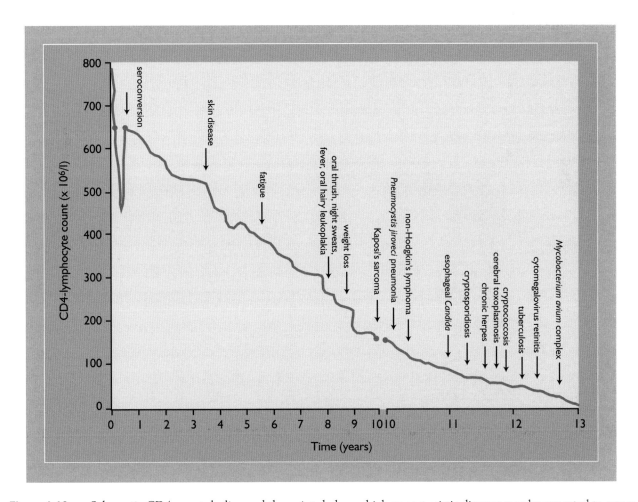

Figure 1.12   Schematic CD4 count decline and the points below which opportunistic diseases may be expected to occur

cardiovascular disease and drug-related toxicities. In such circumstances, AIDS deaths usually occur in those people who have not regularly attended for medical care and are presenting with advanced HIV disease.

A new manifestation of opportunistic infection has been described in patients commencing HAART. Immune reconstitution disease may cause severe, if temporary, clinical illness as the immune system recovers, with acute symptoms of MAC, tuberculosis, hepatitis B, CMV retinitis and herpes zoster and simplex.

A significant number of people on treatment also suffer from drug toxicity. Metabolic complications of HAART, such as ischemic heart disease and diabetes, are a potential problem in HIV practice in the developed world. More patients are also surviving to manifest the symptoms associated with chronic infections such as hepatitis B and C.

Where access to funding for health care is limited, much may still be done for patients infected with HIV. Although the primary strategy should be preventive, significant benefit can be obtained by treating HIV-infected individuals for opportunistic infections, notably tuberculosis, even without HAART. Simple (and inexpensive) primary or secondary prophylaxis for other opportunistic infections such as *Pneumocystis jiroveci* pneumonia

(PCP), toxoplasmosis, MAC, bacterial infections and cryptococcosis may also improve morbidity and mortality.

HIV SEROCONVERSION

Primary HIV-1 infection is often symptomatic, although the non-specific features are almost always self-limiting. Typically, seroconversion may mimic glandular fever, but occasionally gastrointestinal disease or acute meningoencephalitis can predominate. Rashes occur in up to 50% of patients. The most common is a symmetrical macular or maculopapular rash, but it may also be vesicular, pustular or urticarial (Figures 1.13 and 1.14). Sore throat and retro-orbital pain are common complaints. These are usually associated with pharyngeal erythema and edema. Mucocutaneous ulceration of the mouth (Figure 1.15), esophagus, anus or penis is also common. HIV particles have been isolated from these ulcers. Ulcers are usually small, well demarcated and self-limiting. HIV-1 seroconversion should be considered in anyone presenting with fever and a history of recent possible HIV exposure (Figure 1.16). Symptoms last 1–4 weeks. A quicker onset (within 3 weeks of infection) and more prolonged seroconversion illness (duration

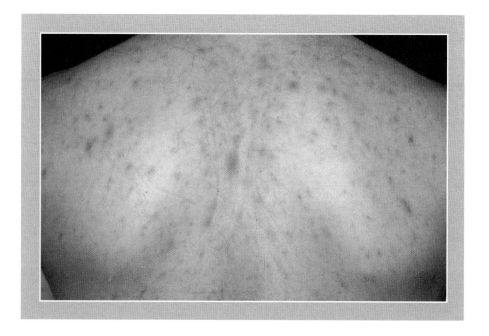

Figure 1.13   Symmetrical maculopapular rash of HIV seroconversion

Figure 1.14   Maculopapular rash (detail)

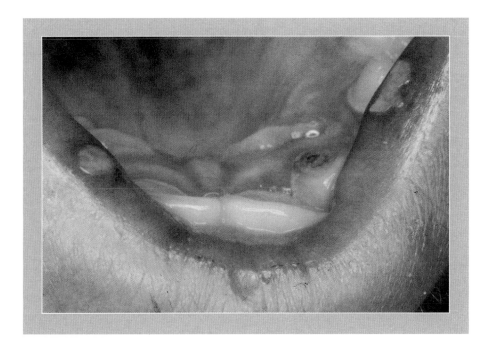

Figure 1.15   Mucocutaneous ulceration of the mouth

> 2 weeks) are associated with rapid progression to AIDS. Rarely, the transient immune suppression occurring at this time may result in either opportunist infections (e.g. esophageal *Candida*) or bacterial pneumonias (in injecting drug users).

PERSISTENT GENERALIZED LYMPHADENOPATHY

Following seroconversion, a proportion of HIV-infected people will have persistent symmetrical lymphadenopathy (Figure 1.17). There is no difference in prognosis between this group and

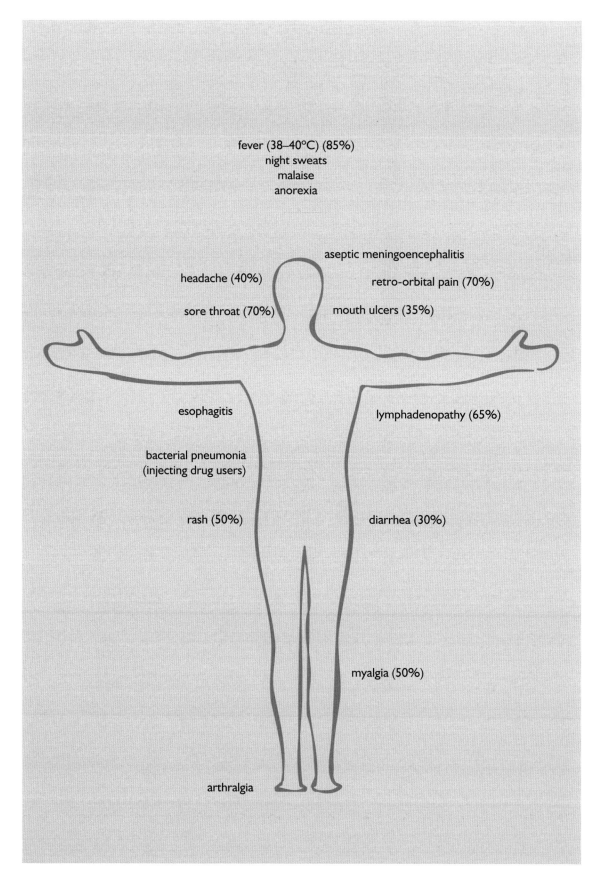

fever (38–40°C) (85%)
night sweats
malaise
anorexia

aseptic meningoencephalitis

headache (40%)

retro-orbital pain (70%)

sore throat (70%)

mouth ulcers (35%)

esophagitis

lymphadenopathy (65%)

bacterial pneumonia
(injecting drug users)

rash (50%)

diarrhea (30%)

myalgia (50%)

arthralgia

Figure 1.16   Diagrammatic representation of the manifestations of HIV seroconversion (percentages given for the most common features)

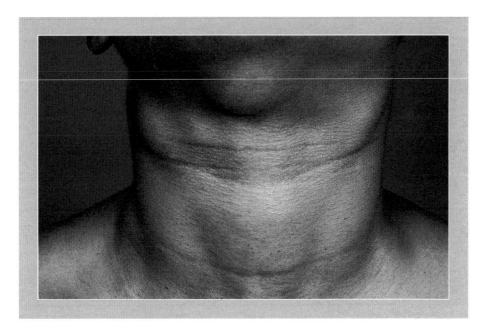

Figure 1.17   Persistent generalized lymphadenopathy

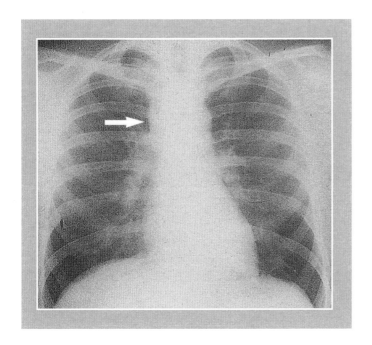

Figure 1.18   Mediastinal lymphadenopathy – paratracheal lymph nodes (arrow)

asymptomatic HIV-positives. Persistent generalized lymphadenopathy (PGL) is defined as lymphadenopathy in more than two extra-inguinal sites present for more than 3 months. The usual sites of PGL are posterior cervical, submandibular, axillary and inguinal and tend to be 1–2 cm in diameter. Lymphadenopathy may also occur with disease due to opportunist infection (e.g. mycobacteria) or tumor (e.g. lymphoma or Kaposi's syndrome) and indications for investigation include:

(1) Rapidly enlarging or painful nodes;

(2) Markedly asymmetrical nodes;

(3) Development of lymph nodes associated with systemic symptoms (e.g. fevers, night sweats, weight loss).

Mediastinal lymphadenopathy (Figure 1.18) is unlikely to be due to PGL and should be investigated. The same applies to abdominal lymph

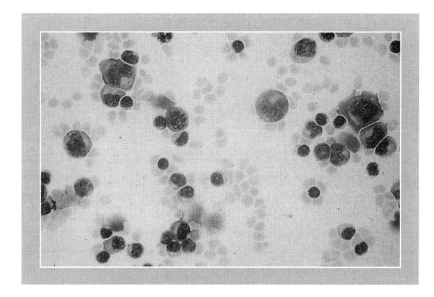

Figure 1.19 Reactive plasmacytosis (MGG stain)

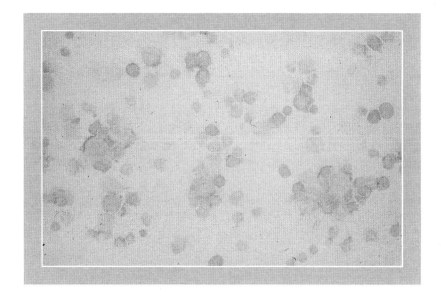

Figure 1.20 Polymorphic reactive plasmacytosis; κ-light chain staining (Dako)

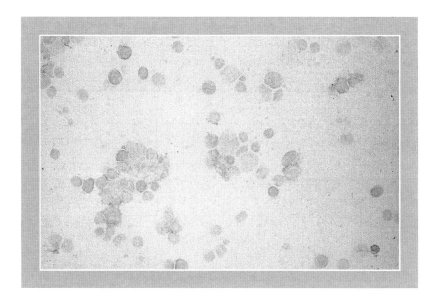

Figure 1.21 Polymorphic reactive plasmacytosis; λ-light chain staining (Dako)

nodes > 1.5 cm in size. Fine-needle aspiration cytology is a useful first-line investigation, and can be performed at the bedside. Figures 1.19–1.21 demonstrate the cytological features of PGL. There is a polymorphic reactive plasmacytosis which shows both λ- (Figure 1.21) and κ- (Figure 1.20) light chain staining. This demonstrates the polyclonal nature of HIV-reactive hyperplasia.

FEVER

Fever may occur throughout HIV infection. Appropriate investigation of fever depends upon the patient's stage of disease, the characteristics of the fever and the presence or absence of other symptoms. In patients with relatively well-preserved CD4 counts, fever is usually due to acute infection (e.g. chest infections or sinusitis).

Major opportunistic infections or malignancies are the main causes of prolonged fever in patients with low CD4 counts. A proportion of fevers may be due to drug reactions, while HIV itself appears to promote a persistently elevated body temperature in a number of patients. About 20% of fevers in patients with AIDS are idiopathic and disappear without treatment within a few weeks. Investigations should be appropriate to exclude the most common diseases (e.g. mycobacterial disease, CMV, PCP and lymphoma). These include:

(1) Documentation of fever with a temperature chart;

(2) Chest radiography and oxygen saturations by pulse oximetry;

(3) Blood, sputum, urine and stool cultures for bacterial, mycobacterial, fungal and viral pathogens (including molecular amplification techniques, e.g. PCR);

(4) Consideration of computed tomography (CT) scans of the head and lumbar puncture to exclude encephalomeningeal disease;

(5) Consideration of CT scans of the thorax and abdomen, in particular looking for pulmonary nodules and mediastinal or abdominal lymphadenopathy;

(6) Liver, lymph node and bone marrow biopsies should be considered if other investigations are non-conclusive.

Disseminated mycobacterial disease (both tuberculosis and others such as MAC) is responsible for up to 50% of cases of prolonged fever. The organisms can be detected within several days of incubation using radiometric broth systems, or within several hours using genome-based diagnostic assays. However, the site of MAC isolation is important as both the gut and respiratory tract may be colonized without causing opportunist disease. Therefore, diagnosis requires culture from a normally sterile site such as blood or bone marrow. There is evidence that MAC cultured from patients with very low CD4 counts in sites other than blood or bone marrow may presage disseminated disease. However, cultures from non-sterile sites should still be interpreted with caution. Figure 1.22 shows an ill-defined mycobacterial granuloma in hemopoietic marrow from a patient with fever of unknown origin.

Serological evidence of previous cytomegalovirus infection is seen in up to 95% of the HIV-infected population. CMV can reactivate and cause local and systemic symptoms. While CMV disease has become less common in the age of HAART, it remains a significant clinical problem. In addition, as already described, patients commencing HAART may undergo immune reactivation of CMV. The diagnosis should ideally be based on virus detection at the site of clinical symptoms. However, CMV viremia associated with fever should prompt further examination and investigation to exclude disseminated CMV infection. A CMV-positive result is predictive for development of CMV disease; more than 80% of patients with CMV retinitis are CMV PCR-positive at the time of diagnosis.

Figure 1.23 shows a typical CMV cytopathic effect in a human embryo lung (HEL) cell monolayer 20 days after inoculation with a sample from an esophageal ulcer. This technique remains the 'gold standard' for CMV diagnosis, although it is being superseded by PCR.

Techniques for rapid diagnosis allow early initiation of anti-CMV therapy. These include the detection of viral early antigen by fluoroscein-labelled monoclonal antibodies directed against the CMV nuclear protein pp65, following 24-h culture of infected samples in HEL cells (Figure 1.24). Histological changes within tissue, such as 'owl's eye'

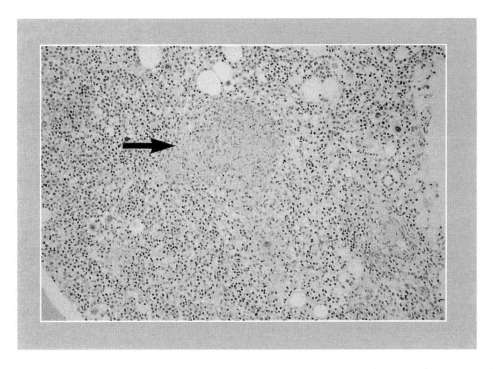

Figure 1.22   Bone marrow trephine (H&E stain). An ill-defined tuberculosis granuloma in a hemopoietic bone marrow from a patient with fever of unknown origin

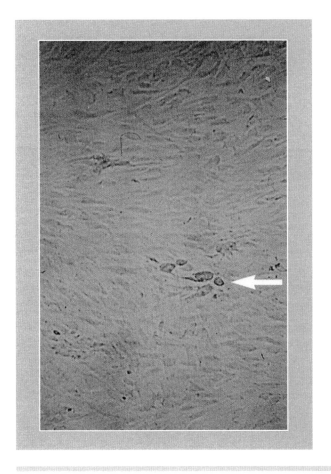

Figure 1.23   Typical CMV cytopathic effect (arrow) in a human embryo lung cell monolayer 20 days after inoculation with a sample from an esophageal ulcer

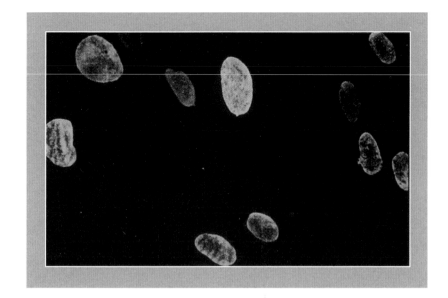

Figure 1.24 Detection of viral early antigen by fluorescein-labelled monoclonal antibodies, following 24-h culture of infected samples in human embryo lung cells

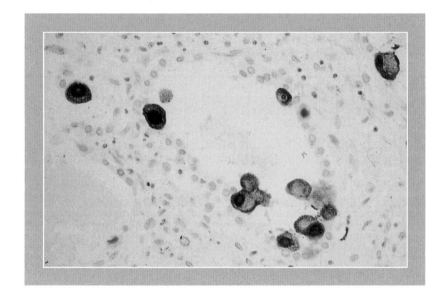

Figure 1.25 Confirmation of CMV by immunocytochemistry (Dako) using monoclonal antibodies directed against CMV antigens

intranuclear inclusions, can be non-specific. CMV should be confirmed, therefore, by immunocytochemistry using monoclonal antibodies directed against CMV antigens (Figure 1.25) or by PCR. CMV DNA may be isolated in blood, cerebrospinal fluid, urine or tissue biopsies.

BLOOD DISEASE

Anemia is the most common hematological abnormality found in HIV infection. Up to 80% of patients with symptomatic disease will become anemic. This is often accompanied by granulocytopenia which is usually less clinically significant. Figure 1.26 (a and b) are the blood films

of a patient on antiretrovirals including zidovudine. He is anemic and has anisocytosis with fragments and macrocytes on his film. There is also thrombocytopenia present, although in general this can be seen independent of anemia and is an early marker of disease. Figure 1.26c shows a normal film for comparison. Cytopenias predominantly reflect ineffective hematopoiesis and can result from infection (e.g. MAC, HIV, parvovirus B19 or fungal disease), neoplasm (e.g. bone marrow infiltration) or drugs (e.g. zidovudine, septrin, ganciclovir, chemotherapy). Zidovudine and stavudine also produce macrocytosis without anemia in up to 90% of patients.

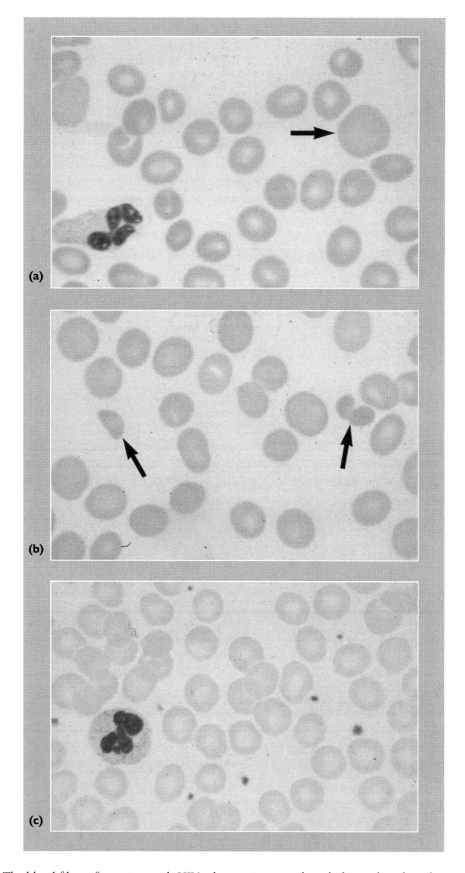

Figure 1.26   The blood films of a patient with HIV taking antiretrovirals including zidovudine showing **(a)** macrocytes (arrow) and **(b)** fragments (arrows) and no platelets. **(c)** A normal blood film for comparison

Anemia should be investigated if the patient has a hemoglobin of less than 10 g/dl (after stopping myelotoxic drug therapy) or has unexplained constitutional symptoms. Bone marrow examination and blood cultures are the investigations of choice. Iron, folate and B$_{12}$ deficiency are rare causes of HIV-related anemia. The severity of anemia is an independent predictor of survival. It also has a profound effect on health status by promoting chronic fatigue. Cytopenias can respond to HAART.

HIV infection predisposes to a hypercoagulable state, with an increased risk of thrombotic episodes. Deficiencies of protein C and S have been reported, as well as antithrombin and heparin cofactor II. Lupus anticoagulant is found in up to 20% of patients. However, there is currently little evidence to support routine thrombophilia screens on patients, although thrombotic risk appears to increase with declining immunity.

SEXUALLY TRANSMITTED INFECTION IN MEN

HIV infection is often associated with other sexually transmitted infections (STIs). The presence of ulcerative and inflammatory STIs can increase the risk per sexual episode of HIV transmission. Therefore, control of STIs is important in preventing the spread of HIV. Conversely, immunosuppression predisposes to chronic and recurrent STIs. Figure 1.27 shows an example of marked penile *Candida* which was resistant to standard topical therapy. Herpes simplex (in the developed world) and chancroid (in Africa) are the most common causes of genital ulceration. Again, they are often florid, persistent and difficult to treat. Ulcerated lesions should always be swabbed for viral and bacterial culture, and dark-ground microscopy and syphilis serology should be performed.

Figure 1.28 shows a painless, primary chancre on the penis. Syphilitic ulcer disease is very strongly associated with increased HIV transmission (up to five-fold increased rate). There are frequent outbreaks of syphilis within HIV-positive populations in developed countries including the UK and the USA. Syphilis in HIV-infected individuals may present with a more aggressive course. Neurological involvement is relatively common, although the diagnosis may not always be clearcut. Vigorous and prolonged treatment is therefore justified. Furthermore, negative first-line serology (e.g. enzymatic immunoassay (EIA), IgM, IgG or rapid plasma reagin (RPR)) may not be reliable in advancing HIV infection. HIV-infected patients may also lose their reactivity to specific treponemal serological tests. Special stains of biopsy specimens

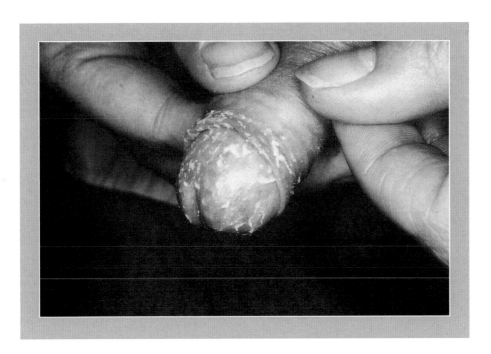

Figure 1.27   Penile *Candida* which was resistant to standard topical therapy

and PCR tests may be required to confirm the diagnosis. It is likely that more co-infected people will progress to secondary and tertiary syphilis (e.g. neurosyphilis). Uveitis is particularly troublesome. Rashes can be atypical and florid, and constitutional symptoms may be greater.

Chronic genital infection may represent severe opportunist disease. Non-healing ulcers due to herpes may need biopsy to exclude other infections or neoplasms. Figure 1.29 shows testicular swelling due to epididymo-orchitis. Tuberculous disease or lymphoma may present in a similar manner.

It is now clear that human papilloma viruses (HPVs) infecting the anal canal may induce the same tendency to intraepithelial neoplasia and malignancy as in the female cervix. Although HPV is sexually transmitted, anal cancer can occur in people with no history of receptive anal intercourse. It may take some years to develop and the current increased incidence of anal cancer in HIV-positive men and women probably reflects the increased survival time

associated with HAART. Anal cancer is discussed in more detail in Chapter 8.

SEXUALLY TRANSMITTED INFECTIONS IN WOMEN

Monilial genital infection (Figure 1.30) that is of new onset, recurrent or persistent may be the first presenting feature of HIV infection in women. It can be asymptomatic, although it is usually clinically obvious. Other genital infections may coexist and, therefore, a full STI screen, including a cervical smear, is advisable. Pelvic inflammatory disease has been reported to have a different clinical presentation and to be more severe in women infected with HIV.

Viral genital infections are common and can be difficult to treat. Recurrent herpes (Figure 1.31) often requires long-term antiviral suppressive therapy, while viral warts may be florid. Figure 1.32

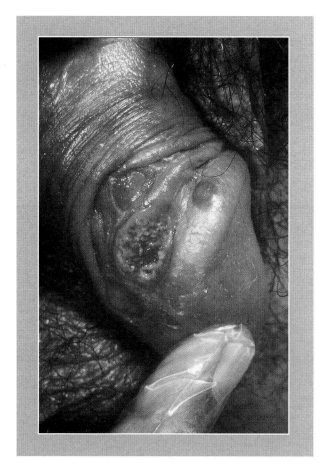

Figure 1.28   Primary chancre on the penis

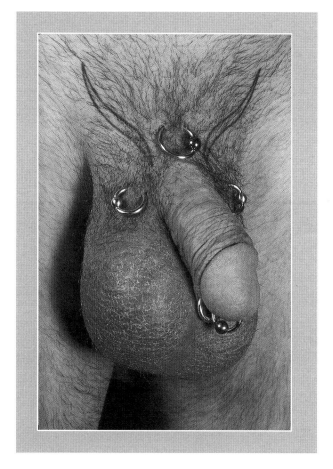

Figure 1.29   Testicular swelling due to epididymo-orchitis

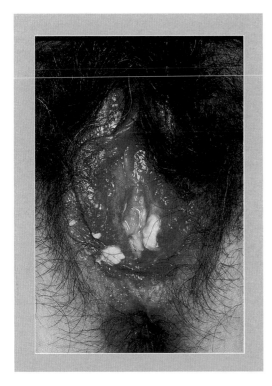

Figure 1.30   Vaginal *Candida*

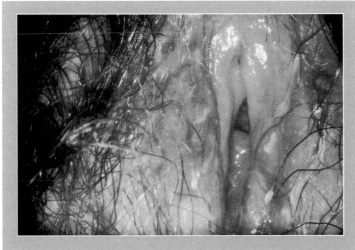

Figure 1.31   Recurrent vulval herpes

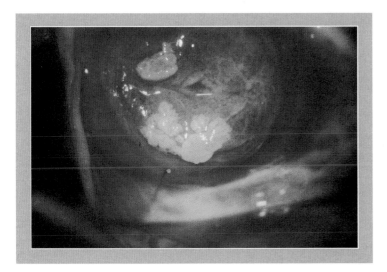

Figure 1.32   Colposcopic view of condyloma acuminata

shows a colposcopic view of condyloma acuminata (staining white with 5% acetic acid).

INJECTING DRUG USE

Injecting drug users are one of the fastest growing HIV populations in both the developed and developing world. There is a considerable morbidity associated with continued drug use. The medical problems that can arise from non-sterile injections include local soft tissue disease (Figure 1.33), septicemia and distant infections such as endocarditis (Figure 1.34) or hepatitis B, C or D. HIV appears to increase the incidence and associated mortality of these conditions. The tricuspid valve is the most commonly affected heart valve, and is usually infected with either *Staphylococcus aureus* (75% cases) or *Streptococcus viridans* (20%). Coexisting pneumonia or meningitis is often present. Injecting drug users who continue to inject do not readily access medical care and will often not seek help until late in their disease. Their dependence on illegal drugs makes them both wary and sometimes manipulative of the medical system. Methadone maintenance programs may be a useful way to engage them in long-term follow-up, and can be linked with a directly observed antiretroviral treatment schedule.

AIDS IN THE DEVELOPING WORLD

The pattern of opportunist infections is different within the developing world. The management of such infections assumes greater importance in resource-poor settings where HAART is unavailable. Life expectancy and quality may both be improved by appropriate treatment and prophylaxis. Opportunist infections are, of course, the product of local pathogens and this is reflected in disease patterns. For example, in Africa, *Pneumocystis* infection, while present, occurs with less frequency than in the UK. Cryptococcal infection and bacterial pneumonia especially from pneumococcus are both much more common. Tuberculosis is the greatest HIV-related problem in the developing world and is the major cause of death among HIV-infected people in Africa. HIV-infected individuals are more likely to contract new tuberculosis and to reactivate old disease. Treatment, when available, is effective, although some drugs such as thiacetazone are associated with a high incidence of cutaneous adverse reactions.

Kaposi's sarcoma has moved from an endemic to an epidemic aggressive disease which is often widely disseminated (Figure 1.35).

Wasting with diarrhea was one of the first recognized features of HIV infection in Africa. It probably arises from infection with the protozoa *Cryptosporidium*, *Isospora* or Microsporidia species.

The effectiveness of trimethoprim/sulfa-methoxazole (co-trimoxazole) in preventing infection has been well documented. Availability and low cost make these a viable option for individuals in the developing world. WHO/UNAIDS is recommending widespread use of this prophylactic to prolong the lives of HIV-infected individuals in developing countries. Co-trimoxazole significantly reduces death and hospital admissions even when patients are also infected with tuberculosis. Hospital admissions for enteritis due to isosporiasis, non-typhoid salmonellas and septicemia are also reduced.

There have been various political and economic moves to make antiretrovirals more widely available in poorer countries. While this is a laudable ambition, the consequences of widespread prescribing of HAART remain to be seen in conditions where there are few support facilities to monitor treatment response and resistance.

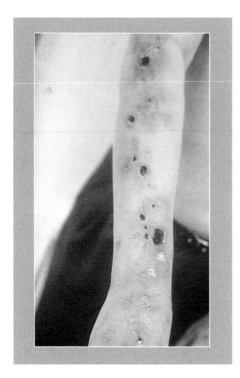

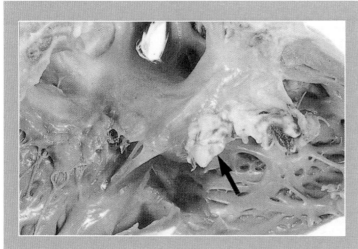

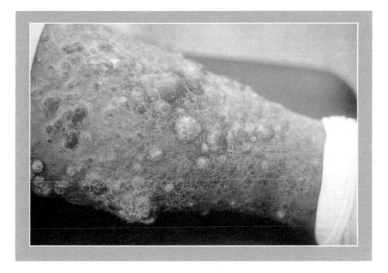

Figure 1.33   Local soft tissue disease on the forearm of injecting drug user resulting from non-sterile injections

Figure 1.34   Acute tricuspid bacterial endocarditis (arrow)

Figure 1.35   Nodular Kaposi's sarcoma affecting the lower limb

2

Skin disease

Skin disease occurs at all stages of HIV infection and is extremely common. However, HAART has greatly reduced the prevalence of many infectious and inflammatory conditions. The associated improvement in immunity may contribute in a number of cases to a transient reactivation of viral infections such as herpes zoster and warts (often oral). HIV-related conditions can be more extensive and harder to treat than in uninfected individuals. The presentation may be atypical, especially in patients with advanced HIV infection. Potentially serious disease often has a non-specific appearance. Non-resolving lesions should, therefore, be managed proactively in conjunction with dermatology specialist services.

Primary HIV infection is often associated with a maculopapular rash, mouth ulcers or urticaria. Pruritus and dry skin, or inflammatory conditions such as psoriasis or eczema, are frequently seen in HIV-positive individuals. Seborrheic dermatitis is reported in up to 85% of patients. The immune disturbance in HIV infection promotes frequent reactions to prescribed medication. Common causes are co-trimoxazole (trimethoprim/sulfamethoxazole), which is associated with rash in up to 50% of individuals treated with high doses for *Pneumocystis* pneumonia, and antiretroviral agents such as nevirapine. Drug eruptions can be severe and even life-threatening. Abacavir hypersensitivity often requires hospital assessment and occurs in 4% of individuals. Stevens–Johnson syndrome and toxic epidermal necrolysis (which can result from the use of several different HIV-related drugs) has a mortality of up to 10%. Patients should always have their medication history clearly documented.

Thinning of scalp and body hair may occur, and tends to be worse if seborrheic dermatitis is present.

Sudden premature greying is also seen more frequently with HIV, probably as a result of malnutrition. Other hair changes include hypertrichosis of the eyelashes, and alopecia (balding). In addition, lengthening, lightening color, and softening of the hair can occur in black people. Medication can cause hair thinning, dry skin and chapped lips (typically seen with the protease inhibitor indinavir).

As would be expected, skin infections and cutaneous manifestations of systemic infection are often found in HIV disease. Herpes virus infections are both more common and more extensive, while persistent molluscum contagiosum or viral warts (often oncogenic strains) are also frequently seen in advancing infection. Bacterial skin disease, usually due to *Staphylococcus aureus*, is common. This can be severe and may represent secondary infection of another skin lesion. Children are especially prone to impetigo. The differential diagnosis of follicular eruptions should always include scabies which can occur in an atypical or extensive (crusted) form. Disseminated disease with mycobacteria or fungi (e.g. *histoplasma* or *cryptococcus*) can produce skin lesions such as papules and ulcers. Fungal infections can also cause yellowing and thickening of the nails. This discoloration can also occur with *Pneumocystis* pneumonia. Medication such as zidovudine can produce brown nail staining.

New infectious agents are increasingly recognized, although, apart from bacillary angiomatosis, most of these have no characteristic distinguishing clinical features. Therefore, laboratory diagnosis is an important part of management. For example, ulcerated lesions should always be swabbed for bacterial, viral and fungal culture. In general, atypical or non-resolving lesions should be biopsied for histological, microbiological and virological analysis.

Eosinophilic pustular folliculitis is a skin disease unique to HIV. Patients typically have a blood CD4 count $< 200 \times 10^6/l$. It presents as an intensely itchy papulopustular rash, often with an urticarial component on the face, upper arms and trunk. Each lesion is centered upon a hair follicle. Skin biopsy may be necessary to make the diagnosis, although it is often suspected clinically, especially if the patient has failed to respond to systemic antibiotic treatment.

Kaposi's sarcoma is the most common skin malignancy in HIV, being reported in 15% of patients prior to the advent of HAART. It is usually seen as a red/violet macule or plaque, although it can present as an area of limb or facial edema from subcutaneous infiltration. Typical local Kaposi's sarcoma need not be biopsied before treatment is started, although lymphoma may produce similar lesions. If doubt persists, or if the condition does not respond to therapy as expected (including HAART which often leads to regression of the tumor), then a biopsy should be performed.

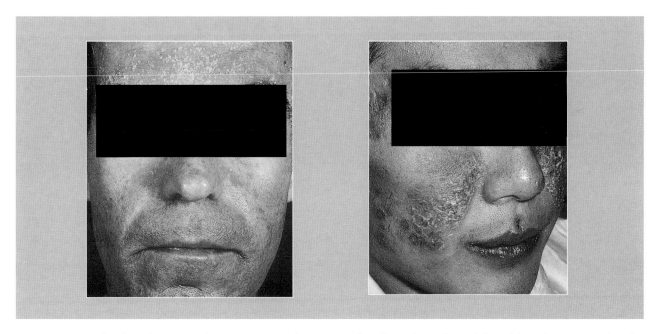

Figures 2.1 *Seborrheic dermatitis* This common condition typically affects the scalp and face although it can involve the presternal area, the groin and the axillae. Seborrheic dermatitis is usually a clinical diagnosis based on its characteristic red, scaly appearance, although, when extensive, it can mimic psoriasis. The etiology is unclear, although often *Pityrosporum* or candidal yeasts can be demonstrated on scrapings. Its severity is directly related to a patient's level of immunity

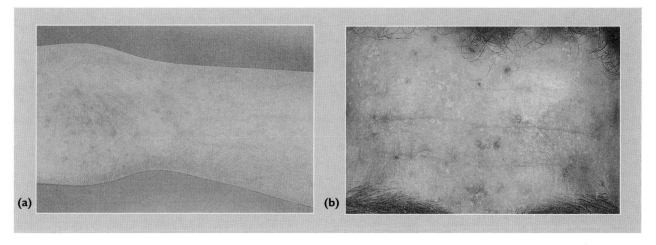

(a)   (b)

Figure 2.2 *Eczema* Inflammatory skin changes are extremely common. There is much overlap between the appearance of infectious and non-infectious conditions. **(a)** Typical flexural eczema with papules, lichenification and excoriation extending up the arm. **(b)** In contrast, chronic severe disease with yeast superinfection.

Dry, itchy skin without apparent inflammatory changes is found at all stages of HIV infection, and affects up to 30% of patients. This may become eczematized (asteatotic eczema) or secondarily infected from scratching. Patients should be encouraged to avoid perfumed soaps and powder detergents, and to keep their skin hydrated with aqueous cream or moisturizers

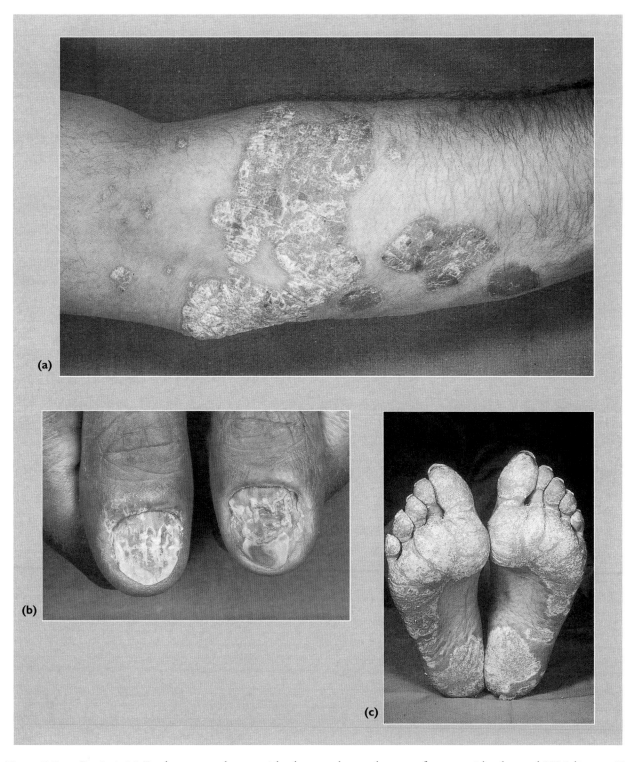

Figure 2.3   *Psoriasis* **(a)** Erythematous plaques with silvery scales on the arm of a man with advanced HIV disease. He had no history of psoriasis, but presented with typical lesions, distal arthritis and nail changes **(b)**. There is onycholysis and extensive nail destruction. **(c)** Extensive scaling of the soles of the feet similar to keratoderma blenorrhagica in Reiter's syndrome. HIV infection appears to worsen previously documented psoriasis and also, possibly, predisposes to new disease. Arthritis is a more frequent complication. Psoriasis may transiently worsen after starting antiretroviral treatment. Reiter's syndrome (non-gonococcal urethritis, arthritis and conjunctivitis) frequently produces skin disease in affected HIV-positive individuals. This can involve the trunk and arms as well as the soles of the feet

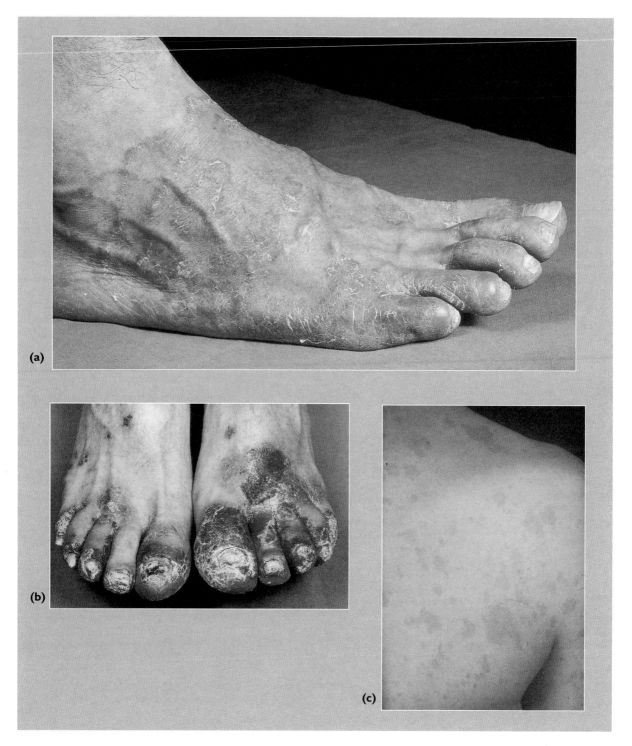

Figure 2.4 *Superficial fungal disease* HIV infection promotes more extensive and atypical fungal skin infections. These are, commonly, tinea pedis **(a)** and onychomycosis, followed by tinea cruris, tinea capitis and tinea corporis. In advanced HIV disease, the typical central clearing may be absent. The diagnosis can be made on skin scrapings. Skin lesions usually respond to topical antifungal therapy, although nail disease will require systemic therapy. Extensive fungal infection **(b)** is often secondarily infected, and both swabs and scrapings should always be performed. Note, also, the severe nail involvement which required systemic antifungal treatment.

    (c) Pityriasis versicolor with the distinctive fawn patches of the yeast infection. The skin scaling becomes more obvious following scraping with a blade, which enables this to be distinguished from vitiligo in a dark-skinned person

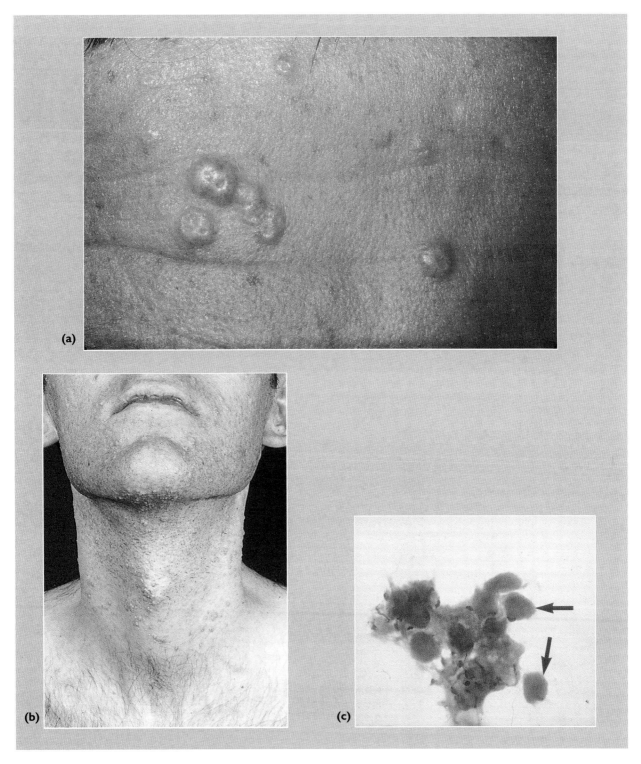

Figure 2.5   *Molluscum contagiosum* Molluscum contagiosum results from pox virus infection. The lesions can either be umbilicated or have a mosaic pattern surface. They are often multiple and can grow up to 1 cm in size **(a)**. They are reported in one-fifth of patients with advanced HIV disease. Patients will usually notice facial lesions, which may become widespread by dissemination over the beard area from shaving **(b)**. Mollusca are more common and less amenable to treatment in patients with advancing HIV infection. They can also closely resemble the skin lesions seen in disseminated fungal disease (e.g. cryptococcosis, histoplasmosis or infection due to *Penicillium marneffei*) and, if doubt persists, skin scrapings or biopsy should be performed. The skin scrape **(c)** shows squamous epithelial cells containing large molluscum inclusion bodies (arrows) composed of viral particles. The residual nuclei of the squamous cells appear as sickle-shaped structures to one edge of the molluscum bodies

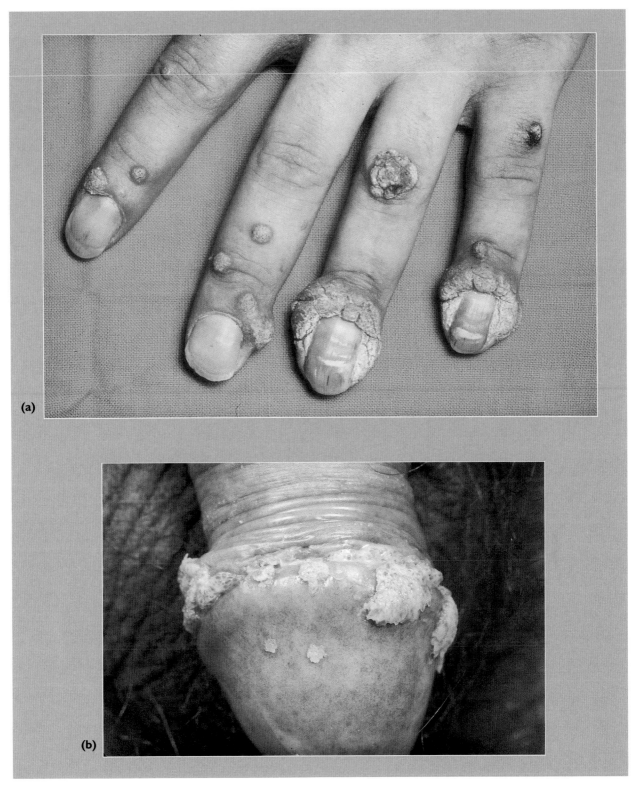

Figure 2.6 *Viral warts* Human papilloma virus (HPV) is a common skin pathogen in HIV infection (overall, occurring in up to one-third of patients). **(a)** The multiple verrucous warts are disfiguring and difficult to treat. This degree of disease is a feature of late-stage HIV infection. The differential diagnosis of a persisting solitary wart includes amelanotic malignant melanoma and biopsy may be necessary.

Extensive facial warts are almost pathognomonic of HIV infection, while the development of florid and recurrent genital warts **(b)** led this patient to seek an HIV test. Genital wart infection is associated with dysplastic skin change and intra-epithelial neoplasia. Treatment and follow-up should, therefore, be more stringent than in HIV-negative individuals

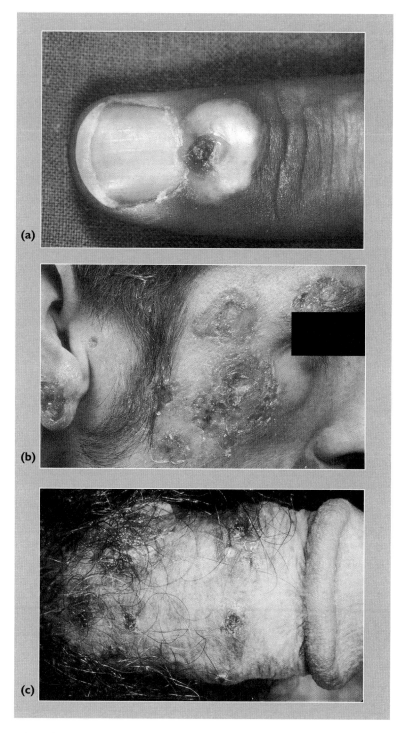

Figure 2.7   *Herpes simplex infection* Herpetic lesions are painful and may be more extensive than typically found in the non-immunosuppressed host. All ulcers should be swabbed for microbiological and viral culture (and, if appropriate, examined for spirochetes). However, in patients with low CD4 counts (CD4 < 200 x 10^6/l) antiviral treatment should not be deferred for laboratory confirmation. Lesions that do not respond to therapy should be re-swabbed (for aciclovir-resistant herpes strains – more common in large lesions) and, if necessary, then biopsied to exclude other infections (e.g. CMV) or malignancy. The sample should ideally be taken from the base of an intact blister or the spreading border of an ulcer. Periungual lesions **(a)** are relatively common. The differential diagnosis includes candidal infection. **(b)** The atypical herpetic lesions were secondarily bacterially infected with *Staphylococcus aureus* and required combined systemic antiviral and antibacterial treatment. Recurrent attacks of genital herpes **(c)** are common and can be reduced by antiviral prophylaxis. The risk of HIV transmission and acquisition is increased in conditions associated with orogenital ulcers. Thus treatment and prevention of herpes are also important public health measures

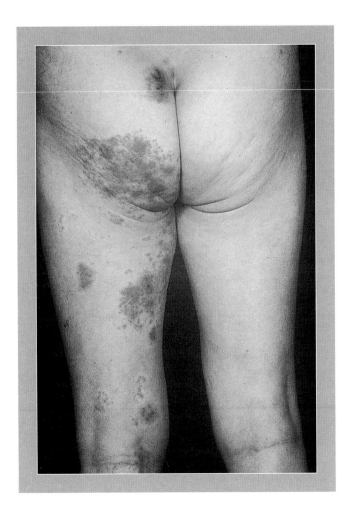

Figure 2.8 *Herpes zoster* Shingles may affect any sensory dermatome but, typically, affects the thoracic roots and fifth cranial nerve. A burning pain or tingling often precedes the erythema and vesicular eruption. As with herpes simplex infection, treatment should be started early to limit the acute attack. It has no effect on post-herpetic neuralgia, which is relatively common in HIV infection. Recurrent shingles is seen in up to 25% of cases and disseminated varicella, as well as atypical ulcerated nodules, have been reported in advanced disease. HIV-positive children with chickenpox are at increased risk of extracutaneous complications such as varicella pneumonia

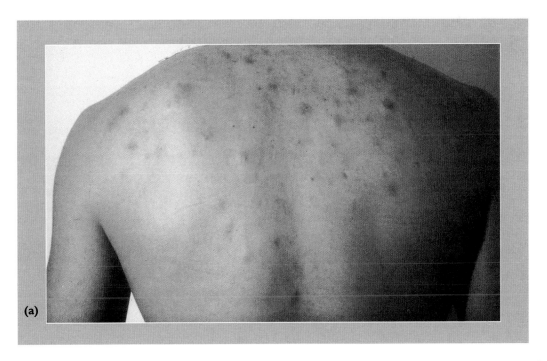

Figure 2.9 *Bacterial infection* **(a)** Bacterial skin infections are more common in HIV disease. Worsening acne is often seen. Frequently, isolated pathogens are *Staphylococcus aureus*, *Pseudomonas aeruginosa*, *Escherichia coli* and *Streptococcus pyogenes*

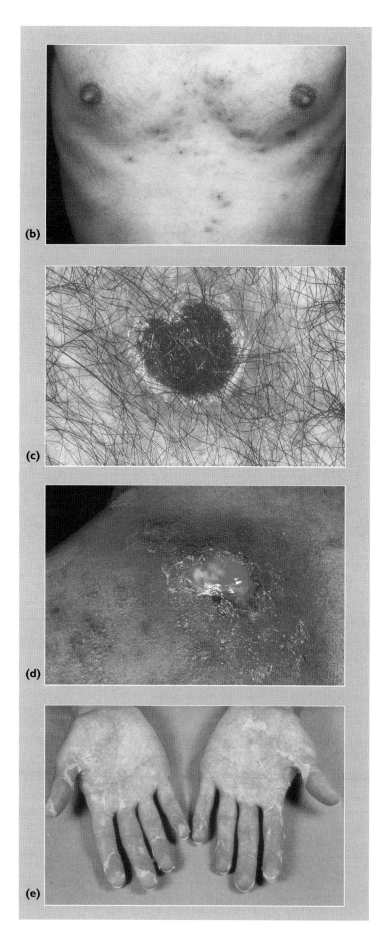

Figure 2.9 continued *Bacterial infection* **(b)** In up to one-third of cases more than one microbial species will be recovered. They may present as a folliculitis, a localized abscess **(c)** or ulcer **(d)**, secondary infection of other skin lesions (e.g. herpes) or as cellulitis. Occasionally, systemic bacterial infection can produce skin lesions, for example, **(e)** the 'scalded skin' secondary to *Staphylococcus aureus* septicemia. Infection of indwelling central venous lines, even with scrupulous skin care, is common, and, usually, also results from *Staphylococcus aureus*. Neutropenia predisposes to pseudomonal infection. With the increasing diversity of bacterial pathogens now seen, it is important that, wherever possible, swabs for culture are taken from skin lesions before therapy is commenced

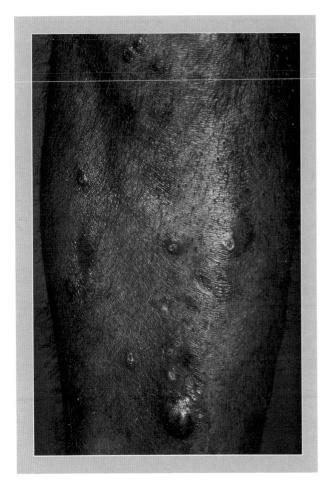

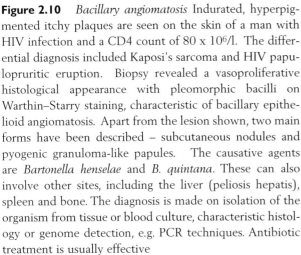

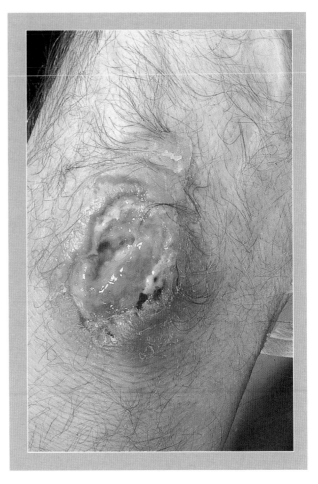

Figure 2.10 *Bacillary angiomatosis* Indurated, hyperpigmented itchy plaques are seen on the skin of a man with HIV infection and a CD4 count of $80 \times 10^6/l$. The differential diagnosis included Kaposi's sarcoma and HIV papulopruritic eruption. Biopsy revealed a vasoproliferative histological appearance with pleomorphic bacilli on Warthin–Starry staining, characteristic of bacillary epithelioid angiomatosis. Apart from the lesion shown, two main forms have been described – subcutaneous nodules and pyogenic granuloma-like papules. The causative agents are *Bartonella henselae* and *B. quintana*. These can also involve other sites, including the liver (peliosis hepatis), spleen and bone. The diagnosis is made on isolation of the organism from tissue or blood culture, characteristic histology or genome detection, e.g. PCR techniques. Antibiotic treatment is usually effective

Figure 2.11 *Mycobacterial ulcer* This non-healing ulcer developed spontaneously. *Mycobacterium tuberculosis* was cultured from swabs and biopsy. The patient had no evidence of systemic disturbance. The skin lesion resolved completely with therapy. Mycobacterial and other complex infections can often present with non-specific skin changes, and usually arise at the site of direct inoculation of organisms

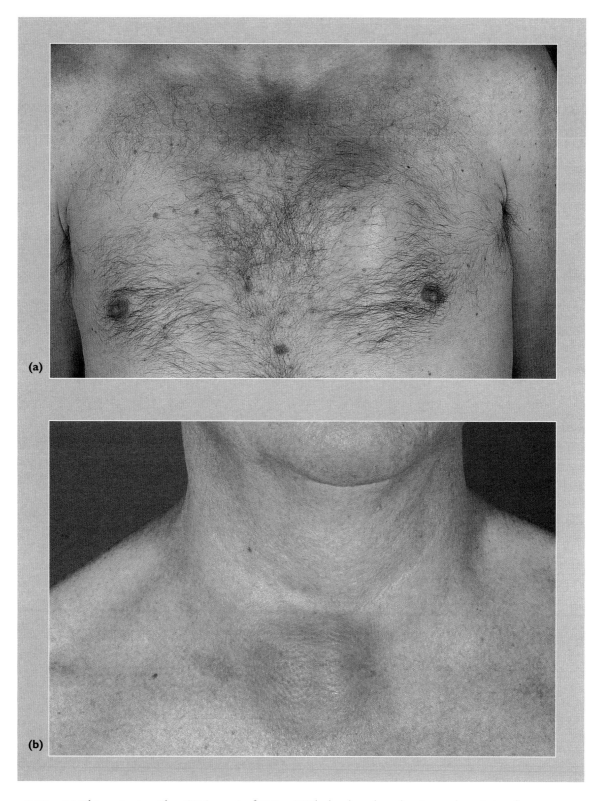

Figure 2.12 **(a)** This patient, with a CD4 count of 150 x 10^6/l, developed a relapsing and remitting fluctuant mass over his left anterior chest wall associated with testicular swelling. He was systemically well between events, but febrile while symptomatic. Aspiration cytology indicated loosely formed accumulations of tissue macrophages. Mycobacterial culture confirmed the presence of tuberculosis. This chronic presentation contrasts with that seen in **(b)**, where the cervical swelling developed over the space of 2 days and was associated with marked systemic symptoms. Tuberculosis was cultured from pus. The lesion fistulated and discharged over several months but responded completely to antituberculous treatment with minimal residual scarring

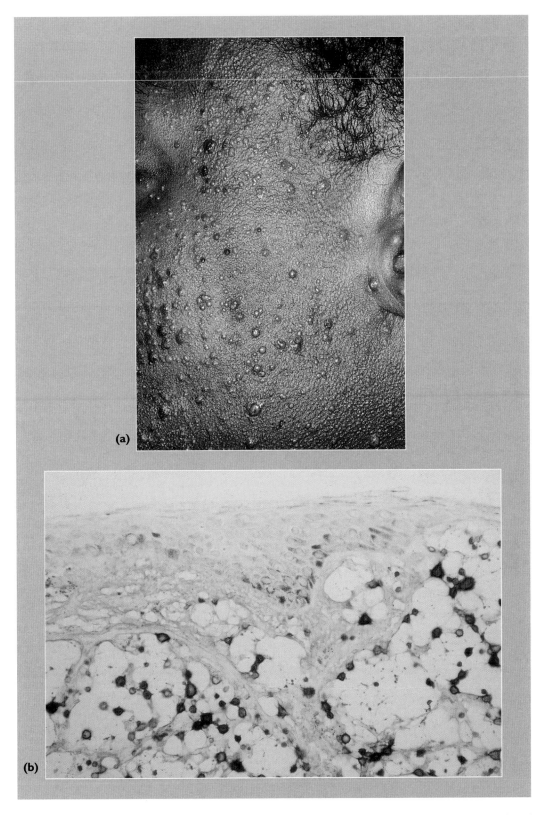

Figure 2.13 *Skin cryptococcosis* **(a)** Disseminated skin lesions on the face of a patient who was admitted with a 1-week history of altered conscious level, breathlessness and fever. He had not previously been known to be HIV-infected. The skin lesions became more widespread, and biopsy revealed cryptococcus **(b)**. This cutaneous presentation occurs in up to 15% of cases. Prompt biopsy of skin lesions should be considered in patients who present with rash and systemic disturbance, as early treatment may be life-saving, and can reveal unexpected, though treatable, findings such as disseminated histoplasmosis, penicilliosis or acanthamebiasis

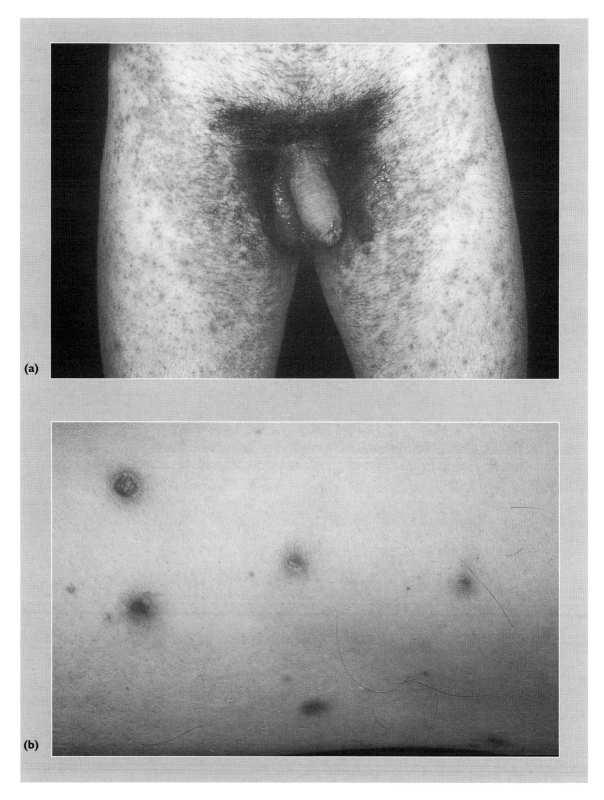

Figure 2.14 *Papulopruritic eruptions* Itchy papular eruptions may result from a number of causes. Up to 50% are due to staphylococcal infection (See Figure 2.9b). Other treatable causes such as scabies **(a)** should always be sought. Here the eruption usually occurs within a month of the scabies contact. Extensive, crusted scabies is seen at low CD4 counts (typically < 150 x 10^6/l), where the mite is able to spread with initially minimal host reaction.

Insect bite-like reactions are common and reflect an abnormal cutaneous immune response. The eruption may be florid or persistent **(b)**. Non-specific folliculitis may require biopsy to exclude opportunistic disease (e.g. fungi) or eosinophilic folliculitis. Black skin appears to be excessively prone to pruritus and chronic papulonodular prurigo has been described

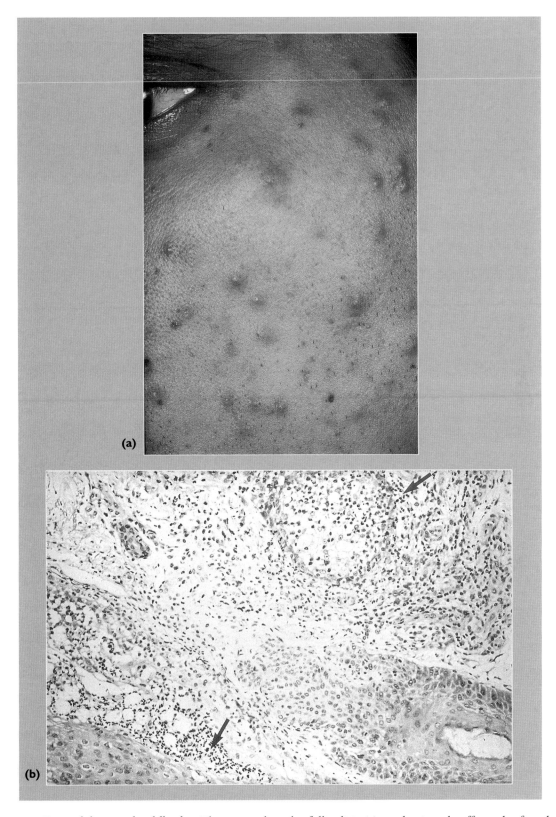

Figure 2.15 *Eosinophilic pustular folliculitis* This intensely itchy folliculitis **(a)** predominantly affects the face, back and extensor surfaces of the arms. The diagnosis is made on biopsy, as bacterial infection can present in a similar manner. The lesions can be difficult to treat. The cause of this condition is unknown, although it is possibly due to a dysregulated immune response to follicular micro-organisms such as pityrosporum yeasts or demodex mites. **(b)** A polymorphonuclear infiltrate comprising both neutrophils and eosinophils within the sebaceous complex of the skin (arrows) is demonstrated in this diagnostic biopsy

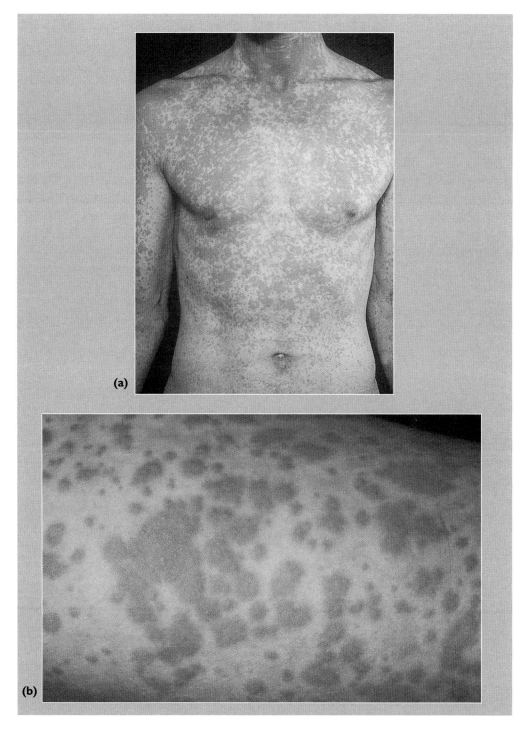

Figure 2.16 *Drug-induced skin rash* Drug reactions are extremely common in HIV infection. They can be associated with systemic upset. HIV-positive patients may become hypersensitive to previously tolerated therapies. Common agents inducing skin reactions include antiretrovirals, antimicrobials (especially antituberculous agents, sulfonamides and penicillins) and anticonvulsants. The patient's medication should always be considered when investigating skin disease. Mild drug rashes do not require cessation of therapy, and, if an important drug is being given for a limited period (e.g. high-dose co-trimoxazole), then the rash can be treated with antihistamines while the drug is continued. Desensitization where a drug dose is slowly increased has been applied with some success to PCP prophylaxis. However, drug reactions may be potentially life-threatening. The non-nucleoside reverse transcriptase inhibitor nevirapine causes rash in up to one-sixth of individuals (with 5% of patients discontinuing the drug). Yet approximately 0.5% will develop Stevens–Johnson syndrome (see Figure 2.17). Women appear to be at higher risk of nevirapine-related rash than men, and it typically occurs within the first 6 weeks of therapy. Its incidence has fallen to 9% following the use of a 2-week induction phase with half treatment dose

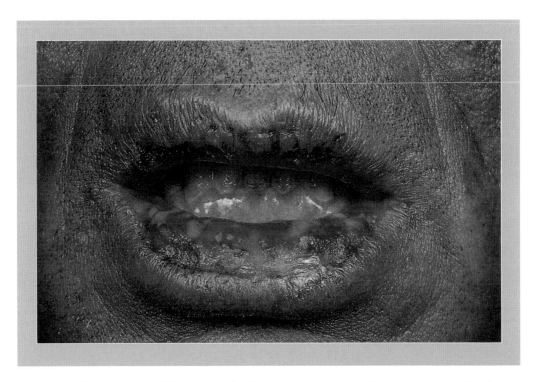

Figure 2.17 *Stevens–Johnson syndrome* This patient developed severe mucosal ulceration associated with erythema multiforme while taking antituberculous therapy. The lesions resolved after stopping the drugs. Ocular involvement by Stevens–Johnson syndrome can threaten sight. The related condition, toxic epidermal necrolysis, is also more common in HIV-infected individuals. The extreme skin fragility of this condition is demonstrated by Nikolsky's sign, in which gentle rubbing of the skin results in full-thickness epidermal loss. This has been associated with antifungals (including fluconazole), antimicrobials and anticonvulsants

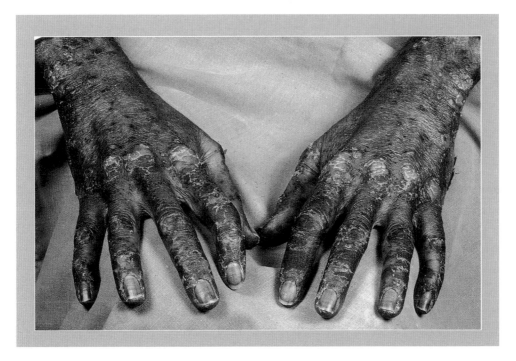

Figure 2.18 *Lichenoid drug reaction* This severe papulopruritic eruption with areas of desquamation occurred after streptomycin administration in an Asian patient previously intolerant of standard antituberculous therapy (see Figure 2.17). The lesions were in areas of sunlight exposure – which is characteristic. They did not resolve upon stopping medication. The patient was extremely functionally disabled by his skin condition

Figure 2.19 *Hyperpigmentation* Pigmentation is often drug-induced and may be associated with photosensitivity. The illustration shows a man taking long-term rifabutin therapy. Occasionally, Addison's disease can produce similar pigmentation

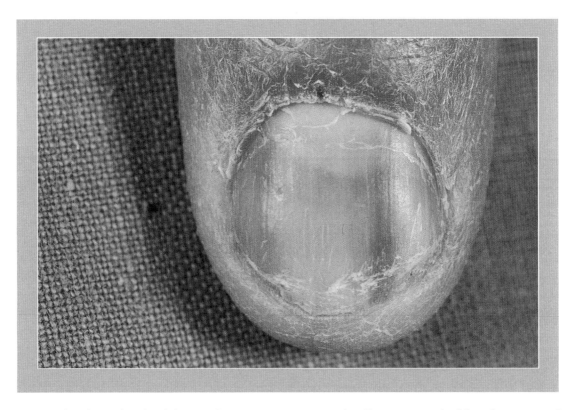

Figure 2.20 *Zidovudine-induced nail changes* The pigmentation seen in this illustration resulted from long-term zidovudine use. The melanocyte proliferation accounting for this often resolves with discontinuation of the drug. Similar mucous membrane involvement can occur in dark-skinned individuals

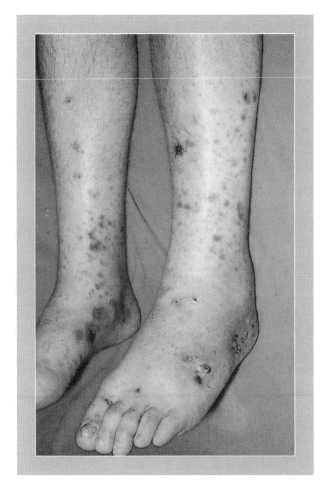

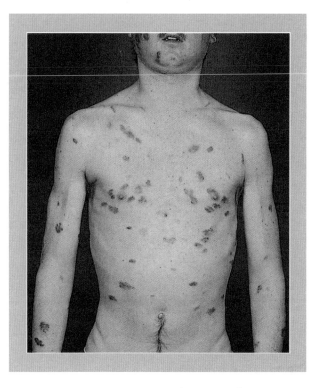

Figure 2.22 *Kaposi's sarcoma* The patient has extensive cutaneous disease. The lesions began as a few flat purple patches on his chest wall. Over several months these became raised and more widespread. He developed facial edema from subcutaneous infiltration. Note the muscle wasting implying Kaposi's sarcoma-associated 'B'-type symptoms, or concurrent opportunistic infection. In its various stages, the differential diagnosis of Kaposi's sarcoma includes pigmented nevi, angiomas, pyogenic granuloma and bacillary angiomatosis. Kaposi's sarcoma is due to the γ herpes virus, HHV-8, also known as Kaposi's sarcoma-associated herpes virus (KSHV). Approximately 15% of gay western males have serological evidence of infection with this organism. Risk factors for this include a history of hepatitis A or B, and increased numbers of sexual partners. It is unclear whether all KSHV-seropositive individuals will develop Kaposi's sarcoma tumors. Further examples of cutaneous Kaposi's sarcoma are shown in Chapter 8

Figure 2.21 *Vasculitis* The illustration shows extensive vasculitis with skin necrosis. This arose secondary to gonococcal infection. It may also occur as a reaction to drugs (e.g. antibiotics or anticonvulsants), systemic infections (e.g. CMV) or as an idiopathic phenomenon in advanced HIV. It represents immune complex deposition in small-to-medium-sized blood vessels. It is, therefore, seen relatively frequently in association with the non-specific hypergammaglobulinemia associated with HIV

3

Respiratory disease

Despite the advent of HAART, respiratory disease remains the most common presentation of severe opportunistic infection in the world. Historically, *Pneumocystis jiroveci*, formerly known as *Pneumocystis carinii*, pneumonia (PCP), was a major problem (accounting for 40% of AIDS-defining illnesses, and with an attack rate of almost 10% within 6 months of a patient's CD4 count falling below $200 \times 10^6/l$). PCP still occurs, though to a lesser extent now that prophylaxis and antiretrovirals are available. Patients who present with PCP in higher-income countries are usually those who are unable or unwilling to access medical care.

Tuberculosis has now taken the place of PCP and can present at all stages of HIV disease. This explains to some extent why it has become so common in many countries even with the widespread use of HAART.

Globally, it is estimated that HIV has increased rates of tuberculosis by approximately 10%. In Africa, 30% of infections are due to HIV. In the UK, tuberculosis is also the leading cause of HIV-related deaths, being responsible for one-third of all mortality. It will infect both adults and children, and HIV co-infection greatly increases individual susceptibility to tuberculosis. The risk of reactivation of HIV-related tuberculosis is between 8 and 10% per year. This is the average *lifetime* risk for HIV-negative individuals with latent tuberculosis infection. People with HIV have a 37% chance of developing primary tuberculosis within the first 6 months of tuberculous infection. This compares to 5% in HIV-negatives. Tuberculosis has been declared a global health emergency by WHO, with an estimated 3 million people dying each year. In Africa, the number of tuberculosis cases is rising by 6% per year – approximately

three times the global rate. It is projected that the annual number of new cases in sub-Saharan Africa will double to four million soon after 2005.

Tuberculosis has a synergistic effect with HIV in suppressing CD4 counts and elevating viral loads. This is most evident early in HIV infection. A large proportion of patients with tuberculosis-HIV will have extrapulmonary disease (e.g. pleural, pericardial, lymphatic, CNS or genitourinary system involvement). Pulmonary tuberculosis may be anatomically atypical – with disease occurring in any part of the lung.

As a result, respiratory precautions are important when managing HIV-infected individuals with pulmonary symptoms. These include a requirement for isolation facilities, with negative-pressure ventilation if the patient is admitted to a ward with other immunocompromised individuals. The use of particulate dust-filter masks by the patient and staff may be essential if the patient is undergoing investigation, such as bronchoscopy. Procedures that involve the production of an aerosol (such as sputum induction or bronchoscopy) should be performed in negative-pressure facilities with air vented directly to the outside. The importance of careful, repeat sputum examinations for acid fast bacilli cannot be overstated.

HIV-related tuberculosis usually responds to standard short-course (6-month) multiple drug therapy. However, patients are somewhat more likely to relapse after conventional courses of treatment for tuberculosis. A regimen lasting less than 9 months was associated with a significantly higher recurrence risk in HIV patients. The indication for prolongation of therapy is persistence of culture positivity after 2 months of treatment with what should be effective therapy, and, possibly, low CD4 counts with no option for HAART, since the risk of reinfection with tuberculosis is high in endemic areas. Adherence to medication is important in all tuberculosis patients. Directly observed therapy can be helpful in maintaining this, when there are issues of possible non-compliance.

Multidrug resistant (MDR) tuberculosis is seen increasingly frequently throughout the world. It is almost always due to inadequate prescribed therapy or poor patient adherence. MDR tuberculosis is associated with HIV infection, although this is probably as a result of the social clustering of infectious cases with both conditions. It is difficult to treat, has a high mortality, and has been implicated in several outbreaks of nosocomial tuberculosis. HIV appears to be a risk factor for acquired rifampicin monoresistance. This may be due to impaired gastrointestinal absorption of medication in such patients. Attention to treatment regimens and adherence should reduce this risk.

Tuberculosis control requires organized contact tracing, chemoprophylaxis for those at risk of reactivation and effective local measures to reduce spread. Chemoprophylaxis should be offered to HIV-positive patients with declining CD4 counts and who have a positive purified protein derivative (PPD) skin test. In resource-poor settings, treatment and prevention of established tuberculosis is an effective strategy. However, HIV infection makes this approach much less beneficial, and it seems likely that HIV itself also needs treating.

The opportunistic pathogen *Mycobacterium avium intracellulare* complex (MAC) accounts for 5% of AIDS diagnoses, and is usually seen in patients with CD4 counts below $100 \times 10^6/l$. Its clinical features are non-specific, e.g. fever, night sweats and weight loss. These are often associated with anemia and an elevated alkaline phosphatase. Occasionally, it may present in a specific organ system, e.g. gut infiltration or within the lung parenchyma. It can be diagnosed on the basis of culture from any normally sterile site (e.g. blood, bone marrow) or occasionally on a blood smear. A single positive blood culture in an asymptomatic individual may represent 'colonization' rather than 'disease'. Furthermore, 40% of patients will have detectable MAC bacteremia within 2 years of their AIDS diagnosis. However, persistent MAC bacteremia is associated with a reduced survival and drug regimens both as prophylaxis and treatment may improve outcome with an acceptable toxicity profile.

PCP typically presents with a history lasting several days to weeks of dry cough, breathlessness, fever and malaise. There are often few clinical signs, although the chest radiograph is abnormal in 90% of cases, typically showing bilateral mid- and lower-zone interstitial shadowing.

Certain clinical features may suggest other respiratory pathogens (e.g. purulent sputum, pleuritic chest pain and focal signs imply a bacterial pneumonia; pleural effusions are usually due to mycobacterial disease or Kaposi's sarcoma). However, dual pathogens are found in up to 20% of patients and bacterial infection (especially Gram-negative septicemia) is now a common cause of HIV-related death.

In someone suspected of having PCP, mandatory investigations are chest radiograph and pulse oximetry (before and after exercise, e.g. 'step-ups' for 5–10 min) or arterial blood gases. Hypoxemia is common in many respiratory conditions and exercise desaturation (< 92%) is a more sensitive indicator of PCP.

Similar presentations are found with viral (e.g. cytomegalovirus, herpes simplex virus), protozoal (*Toxoplasma*), fungal (*Candida*, *Histoplasma*, *Cryptococcus*), bacterial and mycobacterial infections, all of which occur with increased frequency in HIV disease. Clinical improvement after starting therapy for PCP may not be apparent for a few days. Therefore, it is important to establish a definitive diagnosis. This requires sampling of sputum (induced sputum via an ultrasonic nebulizer), bronchoalveolar lavage (BAL; via bronchoscopy) or lung tissue (by transbronchial or open lung biopsy). The procedure of choice is often determined by local expertise. Induced sputum has a yield of 50–80% but a low negative-predictive value, and is easiest to perform. It should always be carried out in negative-pressure isolation. Bronchoalveolar lavage has a sensitivity of over 90%. Transbronchial and open lung biopsies involve a much greater patient risk and often provide little additional information to BAL.

In practical terms, if PCP seems to be the most likely diagnosis, treatment should be started early and a diagnostic procedure planned for the next few days (*Pneumocystis* can be recovered after several days of treatment). In some patients with impending respiratory failure, support techniques such as continuous positive airway pressure circuits (CPAP) have removed the need for full mechanical ventilation. Steroids may be life-saving in severe

PCP. Patients with first-episode PCP and/or a good quality of life are usually those considered for formal ventilation.

Poor prognostic factors in PCP include a long history of disease, presentation in respiratory failure, poor nutritional state (i.e. low serum albumin, significant weight loss), age > 30 years, the presence of co-pathogens and a markedly elevated serum lactate dehydrogenase. Without prophylaxis there is a 50% chance of PCP recurring within 12 months. Primary (for patients with a CD4 count < 200 x 10^6/l, or CDC IV disease) or secondary prophylaxis are therefore important health measures. Prophylaxis with co-trimoxazole also protects against bacterial pneumonia and re-activation of cerebral toxoplasmosis.

Specific treatment of opportunist infections is efficacious. In the first 10 years of the HIV epidemic, there was a decline in mortality from PCP (from 25% to 7% per episode) and an increase in post-ventilation survival (from 14% to 55%). HAART appears to confer a further survival benefit in acute, severe PCP. It has also transformed respiratory care by restoring long-term systemic immunity. If an individual's CD4 count rises to above 200 x 10^6/l and is sustained for more than 3 months at this level, then specific PCP prophylaxis can be safely stopped with minimal chance of disease. The same holds true for other opportunistic pathogens such as MAC or toxoplasmosis.

Irrespective of the degree of immunosuppression as measured by CD4 counts, HIV infection is associated with recurrent bacterial pneumonias. These are usually due to *Streptococcus pneumoniae* and present in a typical manner. However, more unusual organisms are seen with increasing frequency such as *Pseudomonas aeruginosa*, *Nocardia* and *Rhodococcus*. With advancing immuno-suppression, recurrent bacterial pneumonias become more common, such that patients with a CD4 count < 200 x 10^6/l have four times more risk of infection than those with a CD4 count > 400 x 10^6/l.

Respiratory disease in children is common. PCP is often the presenting illnesss in undiagnosed perinatally infected babies. Recurrent, severe bacterial infections are frequently seen. These, together with tuberculosis and CMV infection, are typical postmortem findings in HIV-infected children dying with pulmonary disease.

The lung is a common site of tumor involvement. Kaposi's sarcoma is found in 5–15% of patients with respiratory symptoms. Diagnosis can be made by bronchoscopy, (through the direct visualization of lesions), or suggested radiographically by plain radiograph or CT scan appearances.

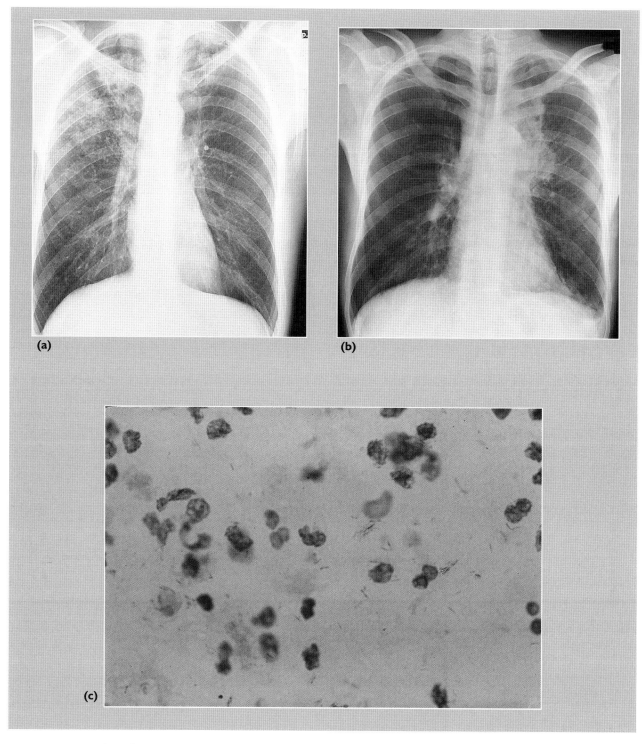

Figure 3.1   *Tuberculosis* The radiographs demonstrate the radiological differences between tuberculosis in patients with and without significant immunosuppression. In **(a)** bilateral upper zone consolidation and cavitation is present, more wide-spread on the right-hand side. The patient had a near normal blood CD4 count. In **(b)** a patient with a CD4 count of < 100 x 10⁶/l has bilateral hilar adenopathy with left upper zone consolidation. There is also some blunting of the left costophrenic angle. In general, there is a good response to therapy; although acute mortality rises with progressive immuno-suppression. Multiple sputum examinations are the first-line investigation but, if negative, then bronchoscopy with BAL should be performed. **(c)** Red staining acid fast bacilli in sputum are seen, confirmed to be *Mycobacterium tuberculosis* on culture. New methods of rapid diagnosis include serological and immunological tests. Unfortunately, they are up to 60% less sensitive in HIV-infected patients, but they hold promise for the future

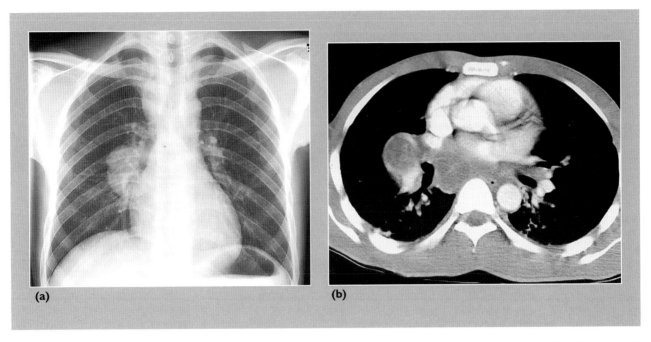

(a)　　　(b)

Figure 3.2　*Tuberculous lymphadenopathy* This 24-year-old South-East Asian male presented with a 6-week history of fevers, weight loss and dry cough. The chest radiograph **(a)** shows extensive right hilar and right paratracheal lymphadenopathy. This is confirmed on the axial CT scan **(b)** which demonstrates hilar and subcarinal lymphadenopathy with central necrosis – consistent with mycobacterial infection. The radiological differential diagnosis includes lymphoma, lung cancer and fungal infections such as histoplasmosis. Mediastinal tumors tend to be seen in patients with higher CD4 counts (usually > 200 x 10⁶/l), and usually do not cavitate

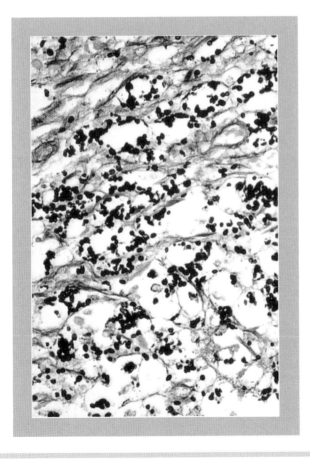

Figure 3.3　*Histoplasmosis* Numerous *Histoplasma capsulatum* are seen in a mediastinal lymph node (staining black). Fifty per cent of patients with disseminated histoplasmosis present with an abnormal chest radiograph, often mimicking PCP. Other features can resemble mycobacterial disease, such as longstanding fever, weight loss, lymphadenopathy and hepatosplenomegaly. Although this fungal disease is endemic in certain parts of the world, HIV-related histoplasmosis is usually a reactivation of previous infection and therefore is not limited to these areas. Like other pulmonary mycoses, (*Cryptococcus*, coccidioidomycosis, paracoccidioidomycosis, blastomycosis and aspergillus), the diagnosis is usually made cytologically, although the fungi can be cultured from BAL or blood. These organisms are fairly common pulmonary pathogens in certain geographic areas (e.g. parts of the USA) and should be considered in patients not responding to standard treatments, or those who have come from an endemic area

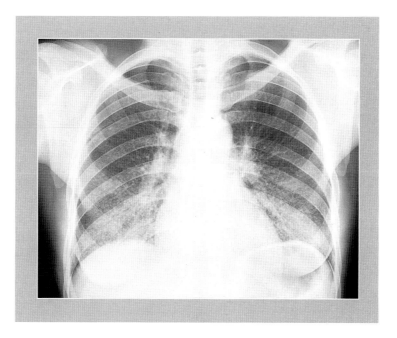

Figure 3.4   *Miliary tuberculosis* This HIV-infected female presented with a 4-week history of confusion, fevers and weight loss. The radiograph shows widespread bilateral nodules consistent with disseminated tuberculosis. MR brain (not shown) demonstrated numerous ring-enhancing lesions. Bronchoalveolar lavage grew *Mycobacterium tuberculosis*. Central nervous system (CNS) involvement is common in patients with HIV and miliary tuberculosis. CNS symptoms may predominate. Respiratory investigations, e.g. CT scan and directed bronchoscopy, can reduce the need for invasive neurological procedures such as brain biopsy. Bacteriological confirmation should always be sought as similar presentations can occur in disseminated fungal and protozoal infection. Classical miliary tuberculosis is uncommon in advanced HIV disease as the poor immune response does not enable granulomata to develop the radiological 'millet-seed' appearance of typical miliary tuberculosis

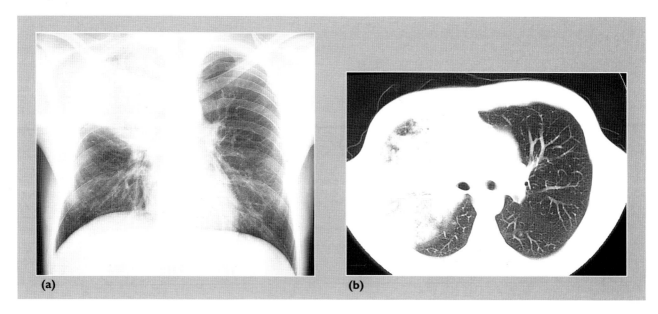

(a)   (b)

Figure 3.5   *Atypical mycobacteria* The chest radiograph **(a)** shows right upper lobe consolidation and associated right paratracheal density. The CT scan **(b)** confirms the pneumonic process. At bronchoscopy, acid fast bacilli were seen in the wash and *Mycobacterium avium* complex (MAC) was grown from culture. There was no evidence of other pathogens present. The patient responded to treatment directed against MAC. Pulmonary MAC can present with a bronchiectasis-like picture. Often the chest radiograph will show non-specific infiltrates. The recovery of MAC from BAL fluid may not in itself be sufficient to initiate treatment, where there is no evidence of invasive or destructive disease, or of systemic dissemination (reflected in a positive blood culture)

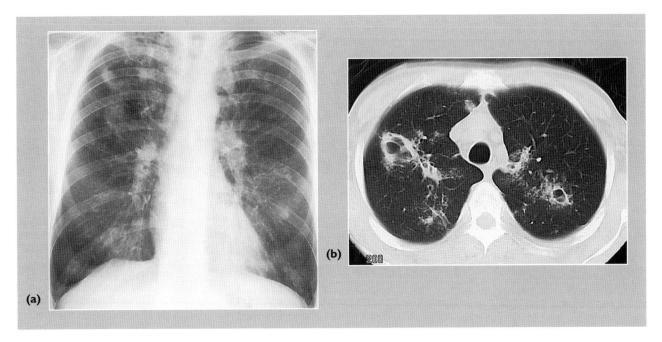

Figure 3.6 *Mycobacterium xenopi* The chest radiograph **(a)** and CT scan **(b)** reveal bilateral apical cavitating disease in a man with a CD4 count of < 100 x 10^6/l. *Mycobacterium xenopi* together with bacterial co-pathogens were isolated at bronchoscopy. Prior to the advent of HAART, *M. xenopi* was associated with a poor outcome and shortened survival. It is now increasingly apparent that this organism is recovered in patients with other infections and that treatment of these, together with antiretrovirals, often makes specific mycobacterial therapy unnecessary

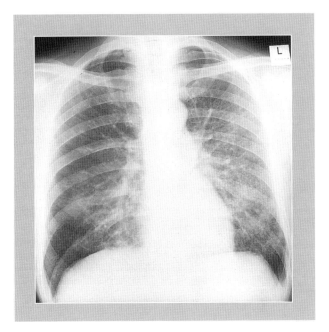

Figure 3.7 *Pneumocystis jiroveci pneumonia* A chest radiograph of typical *Pneumocystis jiroveci* pneumonia (PCP) is shown. There is interstitial shadowing superimposed on the vascular markings with no lymphadenopathy or pleural effusion. The changes are predominantly perihilar and there is peripheral sparing. The taxonomy of what is commonly known as *Pneumocystis carinii* has recently changed to *Pneumocystis jiroveci*. The abbreviation PCP remains the same, standing for *Pneumocystis pneumonia*

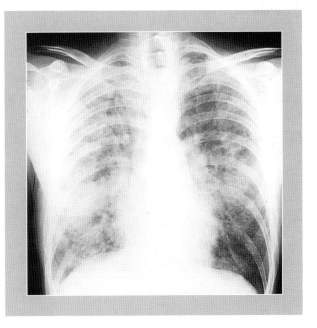

Figure 3.8 *Severe Pneumocystis jiroveci pneumonia* This patient presented in extremis and required ventilatory support for 5 days. He has widespread air space infiltration. While short-term mortality is high in this group, long-term survival is similar to that in patients with less severe episodes of PCP

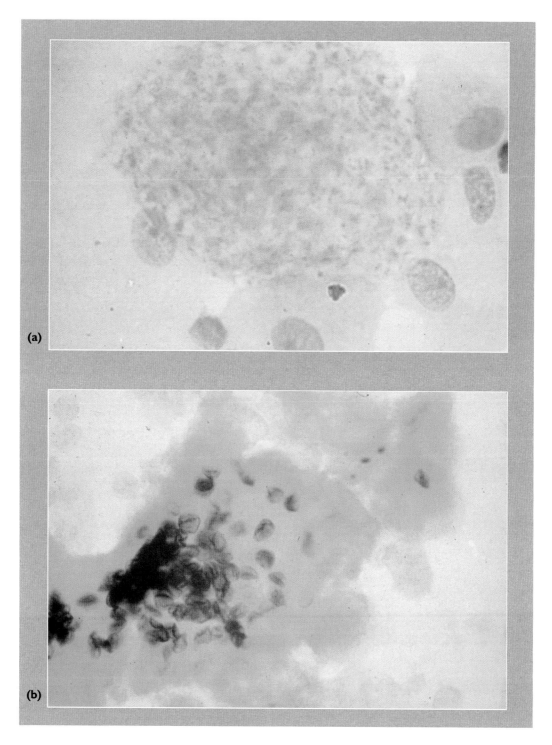

Figure 3.9   *Diagnosis of Pneumocystis jiroveci pneumonia* At bronchoscopy, the endoscopic appearance of PCP and other opportunistic infections is usually normal. *Pneumocystis* is difficult to culture, and PCP diagnosis relies on direct visualization of the cysts in bronchoalveolar lavage, induced sputum or tissue. A number of different staining methods can be employed, depending on user experience. Clusters of *Pneumocystis* are usually easy to see, and more complex and sensitive techniques such as nucleic acid amplification tests (e.g. polymerase chain reaction (PCR of BAL) are generally not required for diagnosis. **(a)** A large cluster of cysts staining purple-blue with several surrounding alveolar macrophages is seen

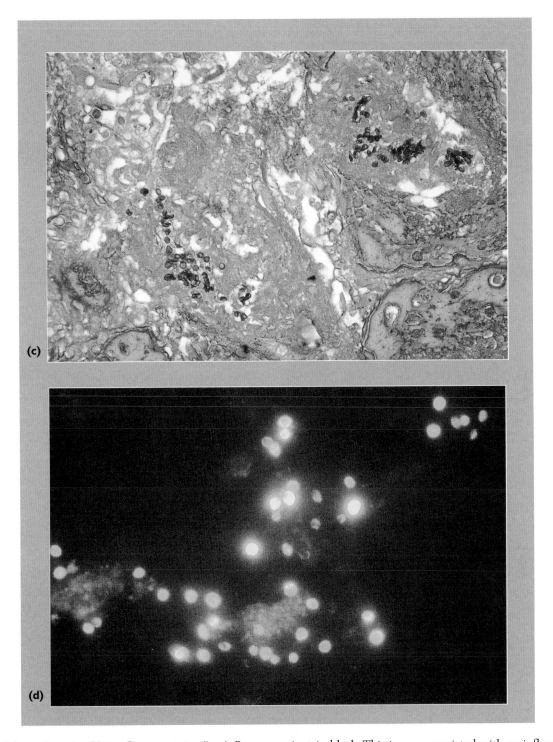

Figure 3.9 continued   Using Grocott stains **(b, c)** *Pneumocystis* stain black. This is seen associated with an inflammatory response, which in **(c)** is filling the alveolar space. **(d)** Immunofluorescence considerably increases the sensitivity of both BAL and sputum induction.

An experienced cytologist can recognize *Pneumocystis* cyst forms up to 2 weeks into treatment. Hence, diagnostic tests can be deferred if the patient is initially too unwell to undergo, for example, bronchoscopy. The use of salivary specimens coupled with PCR may be a valuable rapid diagnostic technique in the future

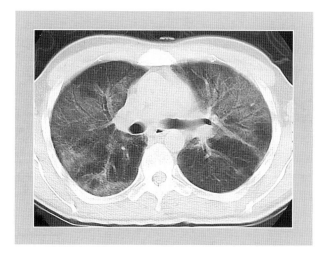

Figure 3.10 *Computerized tomogram of Pneumocystis jiroveci pneumonia* The scan demonstrates the 'ground-glass' appearance of consolidation with relative peripheral sparing consistent with PCP. CT is not a commonly used first-line test but it may be a useful non-invasive technique for investigating symptomatic patients who have had a negative bronchoscopy. CT scanning may also assist in localizing lesions, assessing lymphadenopathy or demonstrating chronic parenchymal disease (e.g. fibrosis or bronchiectasis). Radiolabelled nuclear scanning (e.g. gallium or thallium) is used in some centers to differentiate between opportunistic infections and pulmonary Kaposi's sarcoma

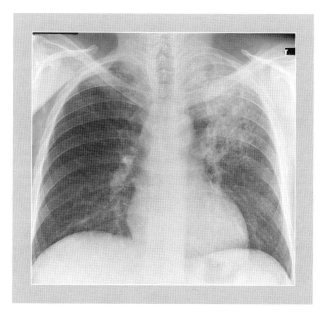

Figure 3.11 *Apical Pneumocystis jiroveci pneumonia* Predominantly upper zone air space shadowing which mimics allergic alveolitis is shown. This patient had advanced HIV disease and was receiving PCP prophylaxis with nebulized pentamidine. The aerosolized drug deposits mainly in the gravity-dependent areas of the lung and thus *Pneumocystis* can manifest predominantly in the upper lobes

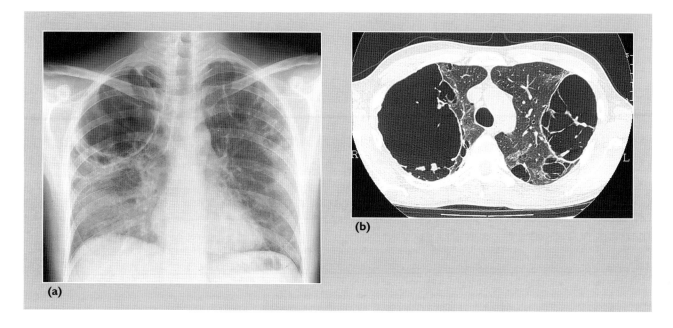

Figure 3.12 *Cavitating Pneumocystis jiroveci pneumonia* A white heterosexual male presented with a 4-month history of progressive breathlessness. The chest radiograph **(a)** and CT scan **(b)** revealed cavities within both lung fields associated with interstitial shadowing. He was noted to have oral thrush and a low total lymphocyte count. Bronchoscopy demonstrated *Pneumocystis*. This can also present as nodular, mediastinal or pleural disease. These radiographic appearances are rare, occurring in less than 10% of cases

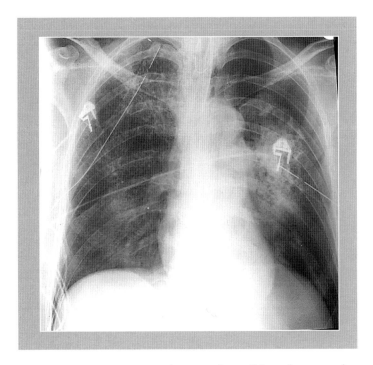

Figure 3.13 *Pneumocystis jiroveci pneumonia-associated pneumothorax* Bilateral pneumothoraces secondary to cavitating PCP are present. There is a pneumothorax of approximately 50% in the left lung, despite a chest drain. Note also a further drain in the right-hand side and cystic lesions throughout both lung fields. This patient presented with a history of sudden breathlessness on a background of slowly progressive respiratory symptoms. This figure illustrates the tendency of PCP-associated pneumothoraces to be bilateral and difficult to treat.

There is no evidence that nebulized pentamidine itself predisposes to pneumothoraces. However, pneumothorax (seen in 5% of patients with respiratory disease) is often associated with either PCP or bullous lung disease secondary to HIV infection. Consideration should therefore be given to empirical PCP treatment in patients presenting with pneumothorax

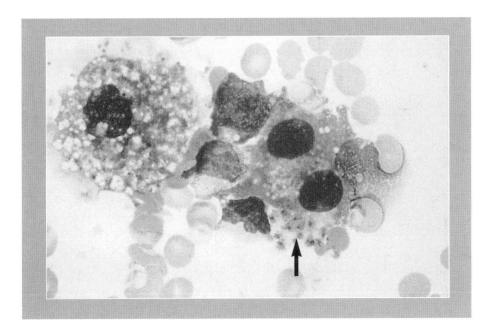

Figure 3.14 *Pneumocystis within pleural fluid (MGG stain)* Pleural involvement is rarely seen with *Pneumocystis jiroveci* pneumonia (PCP), but may occur if there is systemic disease. Occasionally, organisms can be recovered from pleural fluid associated with PCP pneumothorax

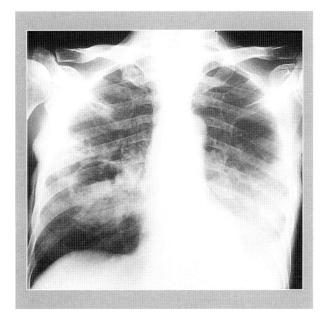

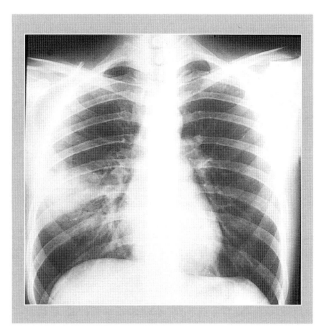

Figure 3.15 *Co-pathogens* Co-pathogens are found in up to 20% of episodes of *Pneumocystis jiroveci* pneumonia. There may be clinical or radiographic clues to their presence, such as green sputum (bacterial infections) or mediastinal adenopathy (mycobacterial disease). The radiograph reveals perihilar shadowing together with a thin-walled right mid-zone cyst from which *Pneumocystis* was recovered and *Staphylococcus aureus* was grown

Figure 3.16 *Lobar bacterial pneumonia* There is consolidation of the lateral segment of the middle lobe in a patient who presented with fever and green sputum from which *Streptococcus pneumoniae* was grown. Pneumococcal immunization, despite its rather limited efficacy, has been shown to reduce rates of bacterial infection and decrease mortality. Its uptake in the HIV-infected population is poor

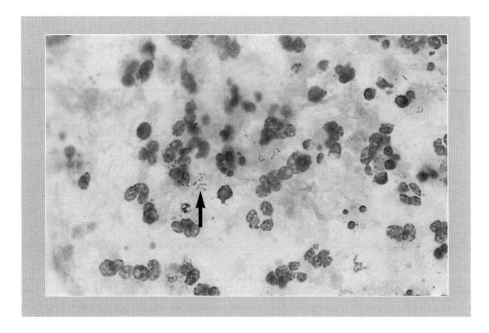

Figure 3.17 *Purulent bronchoalveolar lavage* Pus cells and monotypic cocci are seen, typical of bacterial pneumonia. Sputum culture is a helpful technique if attention is paid to obtaining a good-quality sample. The yield falls considerably if patients have already had empiric antibiotics

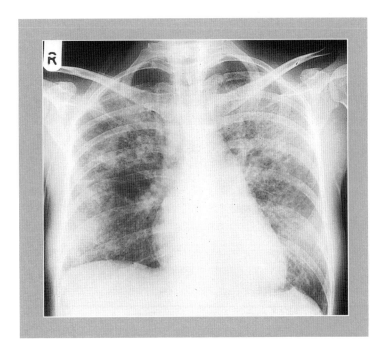

Figure 3.18 *Severe bacterial pneumonia* A female injecting drug user presented in respiratory failure with a chest radiograph suggestive of *Pneumocystic jiroveci* pneumonia. Peripheral blood cultures grew *Streptococcus pneumoniae* and she made a good response to specific therapy. Pneumococcal bacteremia has been reported to be up to 100 times more common in AIDS patients than in an immunocompetent population. Although this figure may be lower in subjects using co-trimoxazole as PCP prophylaxis, blood cultures remain an important investigation in respiratory disease. Up to a quarter of HIV-infected children will have episodes of bacterial septicemia, usually secondary to pulmonary disease

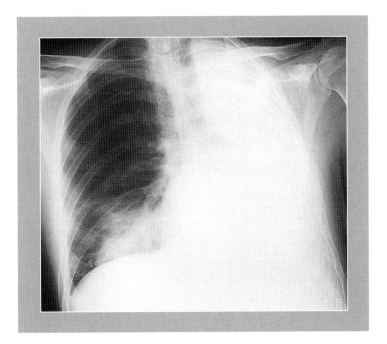

Figure 3.19 *Left lung collapse* A chest radiograph of an injecting drug user with left lung collapse and right lower lobe consolidation. Bronchoscopy revealed distal left main bronchus obstruction from mucus plugging associated with bacterial infection and bronchopulmonary candidiasis. Physiotherapy and therapeutic bronchoscopic clearance resulted in re-expansion of the left lung. Bacterial infections are approximately 10 times more common in injecting drug users than in other HIV-infected populations

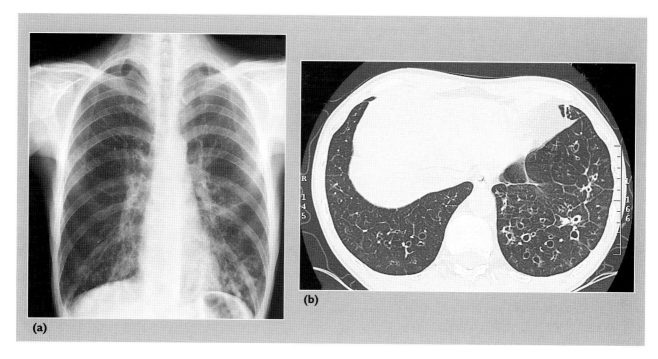

Figure 3.20 *Bronchiectasis* The radiograph **(a)** is that of an injecting drug user who presented with a history of recurrent chest infections and sputum production. It shows bilateral lower zone infiltrates with prominent airways best seen in the left lung. The CT scan **(b)** reveals dilated thick-walled bronchi bilaterally. The typical feature of bronchiectasis, an airway considerably larger than its adjacent vessel, is present. Rapid onset bronchiectasis is seen in injecting drug users. It is also associated with severe bacterial infections. The management can be difficult and chronic sepsis with prolonged episodes of infection are common

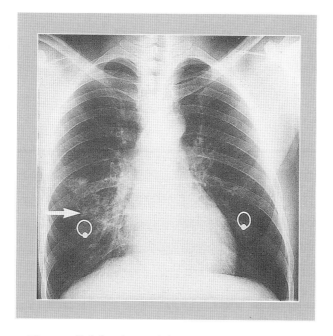

Figure 3.21 *CMV pneumonitis* There is ill-defined consolidation in the right mid-zone extending down the right heart border. This patient with a CD4 count < 200 x 10^6/l presented with a cough and breathlessness. He desaturated with exercise, although at bronchoscopy no *Pneumocystis* was recovered from the lavage. Viral cytopathic effect was noted, however, and CMV was demonstrated on culture. The patient recovered with no specific anti-CMV therapy. Although CMV is often found in HIV patients, the evidence is unclear as to its significance. When seen in association with *Pneumocystis jiroveci* pneumonia, the overall outcome appears to be worse, although there is little evidence to show that specific CMV treatment is beneficial

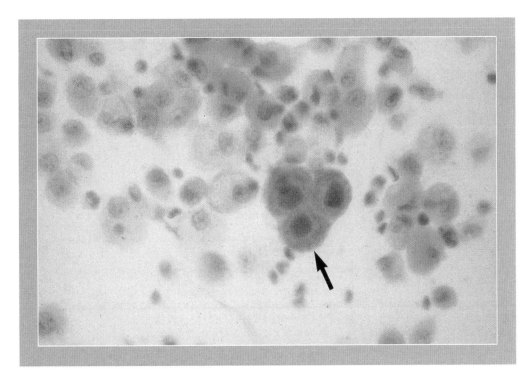

Figure 3.22 *CMV in bronchoalveolar lavage* CMV 'owl's eye' intranuclear inclusions (arrow) are seen within macrophages in a bronchoalveolar lavage

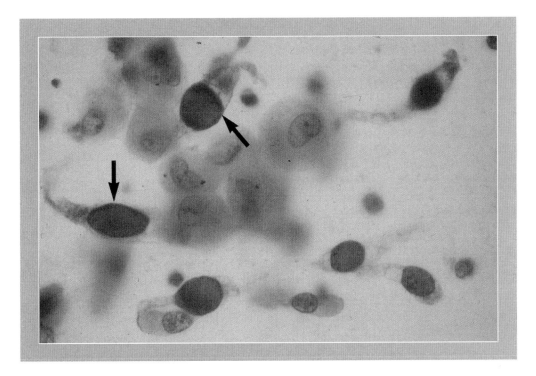

Figure 3.23 *Adenovirus within bronchoalveolar lavage* Hematoxophilic intranuclear inclusions (arrow) characteristic of adenovirus infection are seen within bronchial epithelial cells. Adenovirus is increasingly recognized as a respiratory pathogen. It presents in a similar manner to both CMV or herpes simplex pneumonitis and is usually seen late in HIV disease. There is no specific therapy, and the outcome is often poor

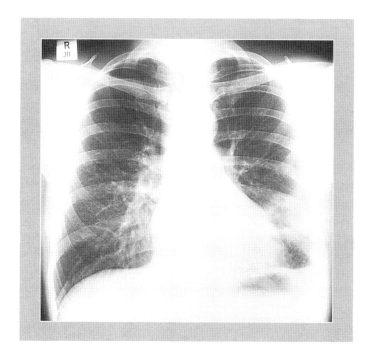

Figure 3.24   *Toxoplasmosis* The radiograph demonstrates cavitating pulmonary toxoplasmosis diagnosed by aspiration cytology. The lung may be the only site of disease, or can be associated with disseminated infection. Radiographic appearances may be non-specific. It is found in patients with CD4 counts < 100 x 10⁶/l and presents with cough and fever. After cerebral involvement, pulmonary toxoplasmosis is the most common site of infection

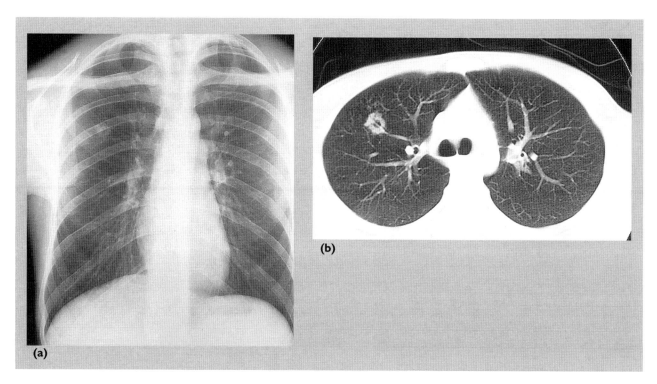

Figure 3.25   *Cryptococcosis* The chest radiograph **(a)** shows a single thick-walled cavity in the right upper zone. The CT scan **(b)** at the level of the carina confirms the cavitating mass lesion. The patient had a CD4 count < 50 x 10⁶/l. Despite a negative serum cryptococcal antigen, his bronchoalveolar lavage antigen was positive and cultures confirmed the diagnosis. This form of primary cryptococcosis is relatively rare, although radiologically it can be difficult to distinguish from other opportunistic infections. Pulmonary involvement in disseminated cryptococcosis has an associated mortality of up to 80%. After the brain, the lung is the most commonly affected site, consistent with its route of spread via aerosol inhalation

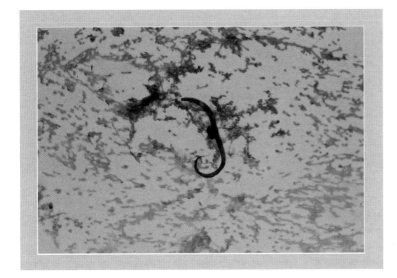

Figure 3.26 *Strongyloidiasis in bronchoalveolar lavage* A female strongyloides nematode recovered from the BAL of an African man who presented with acute sepsis and pulmonary infiltrates is demonstrated. Clinically, he was felt to have a bacterial infection but did not respond to broad-spectrum antibiotics. He was found to be HIV-positive with a CD4 count of $110 \times 10^6/l$. Strongyloides can reproduce parthenogenetically in the gastrointestinal tract of immunosuppressed individuals. This process of autoinfection leads to a massive increase in worm load. The ensuing hyperinfective state results in dissemination. Pulmonary strongyloidiasis, which can initially be innocuous, may be the forerunner of disseminated disease in HIV-infected individuals and requires treatment

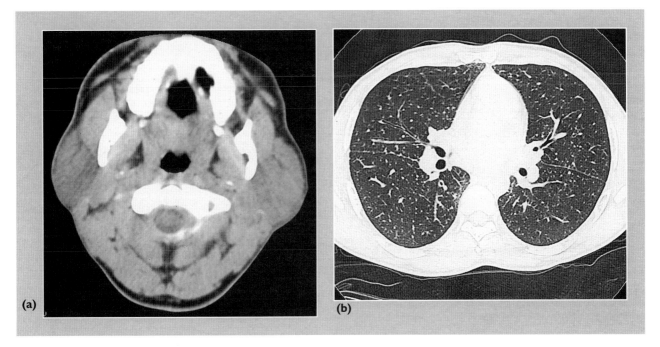

(a) (b)

Figure 3.27 *Diffuse infiltrative lymphocytic syndrome (DILS)* A black African male complained of facial swelling and a dry cough. The neck CT scan **(a)** reveals bilaterally smoothly enlarged parotid glands. The high-resolution CT scan **(b)** of the chest shows ill-defined nodules throughout both lung fields. The centrilobular distribution was consistent with lymphocytic interstitial pneumonitis. This was confirmed on bronchoalveolar lavage where a CD8-predominant lymphocytosis was demonstrated. The association of T-cell infiltrates in parotids, muscle, bone, lung and brain is well-documented. No specific pathogen has been implicated, although there are possible associations with Epstein–Barr virus. There are HLA associations and DILS can occur in subjects with either relatively well-preserved immunity or who have had a good response to antiretroviral treatment. It is possible that a proportion of DILS will transform with time into lymphoma.

Lymphocytic interstitial pneumonitis (LIP) is reported in up to 40% of children with perinatally acquired HIV infection. It presents with gradually progressive breathlessness associated with cough, wheeze and digital clubbing. Systemic signs are similar to the adult form. Distinction from chronic PCP can be difficult, although, unlike PCP, LIP tends to occur in children aged 1 and above. Diagnosis may require tissue biopsy, and bacterial superinfections are common.

Nodularity on CT scans is often due to opportunistic infection. Common causes include bacterial pneumonia and tuberculosis. Often these can be distinguished on clinical grounds, although it is important to obtain laboratory confirmation of the diagnosis

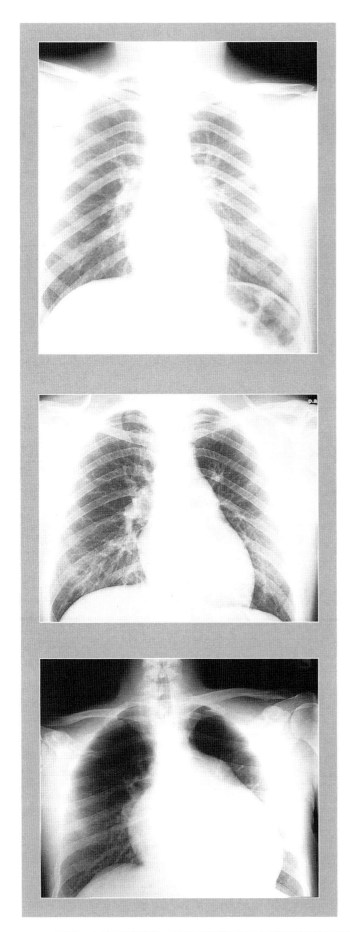

Figure 3.28 *Progressive pulmonary hypertension* The serial radiographs are of a young, HIV-infected male who complained of progressive breathlessness and exercise-induced chest pain. At each 2-year interval there is an increase in the cardiothoracic ratio and pulmonary artery prominence. Pulmonary artery catheterization confirmed the diagnosis of HIV-associated pulmonary hypertension. This condition is seen at an estimated frequency of 1 in 200 in HIV-infected individuals – many times more than in the general population. It commonly presents in young males at any CD4 count. The pulmonary arteriopathy that is typically seen on histology may arise from HIV protein and cytokine-mediated vasoconstriction and endothelial proliferaton. It must be distinguished from pulmonary vascular abnormalities associated with illicit drug use such as injection of talc or smoking crack cocaine. Current treatment combines HAART and inhibitors of endothelin-1, a potent vasoconstrictor

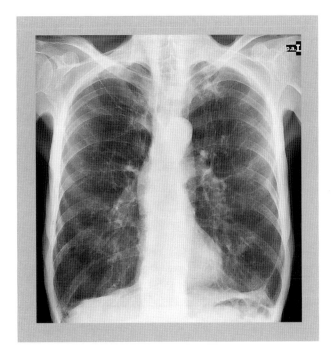

Figure 3.29 *Chronic obstructive pulmonary disease* The chest radiograph shows widespread bullous emphysema in a 50-year-old male HIV-infected smoker. Despite a good response to antiretroviral therapy, he was disabled by his lung disease. Studies have indicated that there is an accelerated rate of lung volume loss in such individuals. Premature bullous emphysema is not reversible. Given the prolonged survival offered by HAART, together with high smoking rates in many HIV-infected populations, attempts to promote smoking cessation should be a priority among health-care workers. Twelve months after this radiograph was taken, this patient was diagnosed with lung cancer

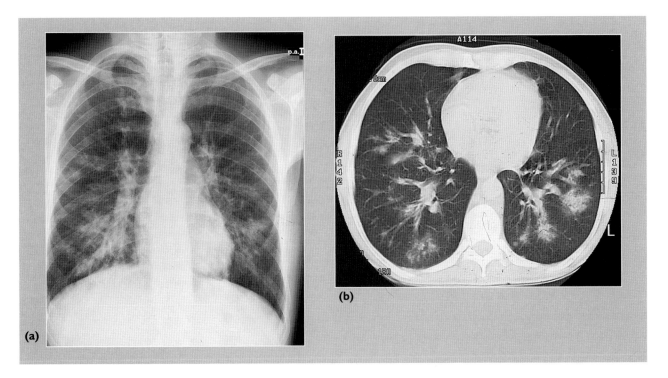

Figure 3.30 *Pulmonary Kaposi's sarcoma* This condition often presents with progressive breathlessness and cough in patients with cutaneous Kaposi's sarcoma. The chest radiograph **(a)** shows ill-defined opacities in both lung fields, predominantly in the mid- and lower zones. The CT scan **(b)** confirms their bronchocentric distribution – characteristic of pulmonary Kaposi's sarcoma. Both hilar or mediastinal adenopathy and pleural effusion are common. However, the distinction from *Pneumocystis jiroveci* pneumonia can often be difficult

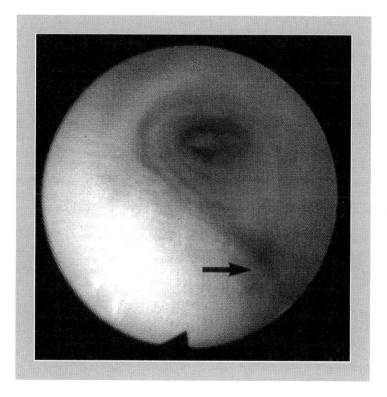

Figure 3.31   *Kaposi's sarcoma* A bronchoscopic view of Kaposi's sarcoma in the mid-trachea. The diagnosis can be made by direct visualization in up to 50% of patients (those with proximal lesions). The presence of hemosiderin-laden macrophages in the bronchoalveolar lavage may support the clinical diagnosis (as this suggests pulmonary hemorrhage)

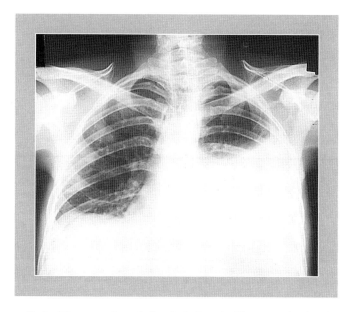

Figure 3.32   *Lymphomatous effusion* There is a large left-sided pleural effusion and subpulmonary fluid on the right. The patient gave a 2-month history of fever, weight loss and abdominal pain. The diagnosis of non-Hodgkin's lymphoma was made cytologically on pleural aspirate. Primary effusion lymphoma has been associated with human herpesvirus 8 (HHV-8). This sexually transmitted virus contributes to the high prevalence of Kaposi's sarcoma. Angiofollicular lymphoid hyperplasia (Castleman's syndrome) is another HHV-8-associated disease which is more common in this population.

Apart from lymphoma, large effusions may also be seen in mycobacterial disease and Kaposi's sarcoma. In the latter case, the effusions will often be bloodstained. Although simple aspiration is a useful procedure, more information can be gained from the histology and culture of a pleural biopsy, best obtained by thoracoscopy. Smaller effusions are usually due to bacterial infection, although in wasted, malnourished patients, hypoalbuminemia is a common cause

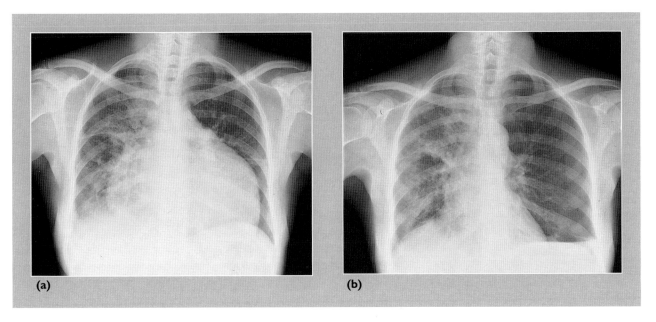

(a)

(b)

Figure 3.33 *Tuberculous pericarditis* An HIV-infected female presented with progressive breathlessness, fevers, weight loss and confusion. The chest radiograph **(a)** shows globular cardiomegaly and predominantly right-sided infiltrates, together with a pleural effusion. The crispness of the cardiac outline suggested reduced cardiac movement. An echocardiogram confirmed a large pericardial effusion compromising cardiac function. Aspiration of 1 liter of serosanguinous fluid resulted in an improvement in her hemodynamic state **(b)**. *Mycobacterium tuberculosis* was grown from pericardial fluid. Tuberculosis is responsible for up to 40% of HIV-associated pericardial effusions. Other causes include Kaposi's sarcoma, CMV, bacterial and fungal infections

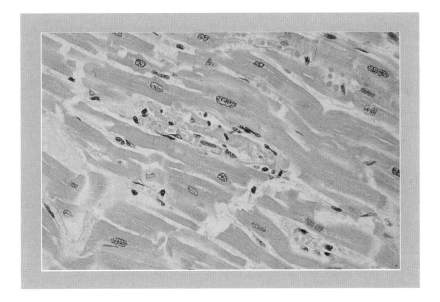

Figure 3.34 *HIV cardiomyopathy (H&E stain)* A degenerating myocardial fiber is demonstrated. This reflects presumed direct HIV infection and is a common postmortem finding (in up to 30% of cases), although clinically it is relatively rare. It presents in late-stage disease as a dilated cardiomyopathy; or may be noted before this as diastolic impairment. It has been reported that up to three-quarters of HIV-infected children had evidence of left ventricular dysfunction and 20% developed cardiac failure. Endomyocardial biopsy may be indicated to exclude treatable opportunistic infection such as toxoplasmosis and CMV. The pathogenesis of HIV-related cardiomyopathy is uncertain. Explanations include an autoimmune response to viral infection and selenium deficiency. Its frequency appears to have declined with the use of HAART. This may explain the reduction in cardiac mortality that is seen in patients on antiretrovirals. However, the lipid abnormalities that occur with HAART may in fact increase the risk of cardiovascular events such as myocardial infarction. Strenuous attempts should be made to reduce any cardiac risk through smoking cessation, diet and exercise

4

Gastrointestinal disease

The common presentations of gastrointestinal disease are oral disease, difficulty swallowing, abdominal pain and diarrhea.

ORAL DISEASE

Oral candidal infection and oral hairy leukoplakia are the most common oral lesions. Pre-HAART, their prevalence approached 50% in the HIV-infected population. They are important clinical markers of progressive HIV disease, indicating a loss of mucosal immunity. Candidiasis may be the first symptom of HIV infection (in up to 25% cases). It is most common in its pseudomembranous form as thrush. Oral hairy leukoplakia is often an incidental finding. Gingivitis and periodontitis are common, and HIV patients should have regular dental check-ups.

Mouth ulcers may result from a variety of causes and should be swabbed for microbiological and virological culture. Painful ulcers are often due to herpes simplex virus (HSV) and a course of aciclovir can be given while awaiting laboratory confirmation. Non-resolving ulceration may result from fungal disease (e.g. *Cryptococcus* or *Mucoraceae*), bacteria (e.g. *E. coli*), viruses (e.g. CMV), drug reactions (e.g. the anti-retroviral agent, zalcitabine), malignancy (e.g. lymphoma) or idiopathic causes (aphthous ulcers). Syphilis serology and dark background microscopy should be performed if the snail-track ulcers of secondary syphilis are suspected. Primary HIV infection is associated with oral or even esophageal ulceration in up to 40% of symptomatic cases. These have the appearance of aphthous ulcers. Oral thrush and sore throat with pharyngeal erythema are other common findings during acute seroconversion.

Up to 40% of all Kaposi's sarcoma presents in the mouth. Its characteristic purple-red appearance is usually found on the hard palate.

SALIVARY GLAND DISEASE

Bilateral parotid enlargement occurs with increased frequency in HIV infection. It may result from diffuse infiltrative lymphocytic syndrome (DILS), where there is glandular infiltration with CD8 T cells. This is part of the systemic condition described in Chapter 3 (Figure 3.27). Other causes of salivary gland enlargement include CMV infection, tuberculosis and tumors, such as Kaposi's sarcoma and lymphoma. It may also be seen in the context of a sicca-like syndrome with dry eyes and reduced saliva production. This has been reported more frequently since HAART was introduced and is probably a direct effect of medication.

DIFFICULTY SWALLOWING

One-third of AIDS patients will develop esophageal symptoms during their illness. Retrosternal discomfort when swallowing suggests severe opportunistic infection usually due to *Candida* esophagitis (50–75% of cases). This may be associated with some weight loss although patients can usually maintain adequate hydration. Esophageal candidiasis is a common AIDS-defining illness, and, in general, should be carefully documented by endoscopic visualization (and brushings/biopsy). The procedure carries little risk of either complications or cross-infection. If pain (odynophagia) is a prominent feature, or there has been no improvement on empirical antifungal therapy, then likely infections are CMV or, occasionally, HSV. The diagnosis should be established by endoscopy. Aphthous ulceration is reported in up to 30% of patients with odynophagia.

Esophageal ulceration may be due to HIV infection itself. This diagnosis should only be made after opportunistic infections and drug associations have been excluded (see above).

ABDOMINAL PAIN AND DIARRHEA

Diarrhea occurs in a high proportion of HIV-infected individuals in both the developed and the developing world. Up to 50% of the former, and at least 90% of the latter will be affected. It occurs in both adults and children and is often associated with severe weight loss and malnutrition (HIV wasting syndrome). In many studies, nutritional status is an independent predictor of death. Chronic diarrhea has a profound impact on quality of life. The introduction of HAART has led to a marked reduction in the frequency of isolation of enteric pathogens. Previously, these could be demonstrated in 60–85% of cases, now it is closer to 15%. The importance of HAART cannot be overestimated as many of the causative agents that are present at low CD4 counts ($< 100 \times 10^6/1$) have no specific treatment.

HIV-related diarrhea results from both typical pathogens as well as opportunistic infectious causes. What should be self-terminating diseases often persist in the immunosuppressed host. The clinical features of the diarrheal illness can sometimes help with diagnosis. For example, watery, profuse diarrhea associated with cramping pains may be due to Cryptosporidia species, *Isospora belli* or Microsporidia species. Dysentery with blood and pus in the stool, associated with fever and malaise, can be due to CMV colitis or *Salmonella*. More often, the features are non-specific. Thus, a stepwise investigation of diarrhea in HIV disease has been developed. This starts with multiple stool samples for microscopy and culture, and progresses to more complex and invasive procedures if this step is negative (see Figure 4.16).

Upper and lower gastrointestinal symptoms may result from gut wall infiltration by tumors such as Kaposi's sarcoma or lymphoma. These can be seen on endoscopic examination.

Severe CMV enteritis occurs in about 3% of AIDS patients. The diagnosis should be based strictly on either histology (inclusions with surrounding inflammation) or culture with appropriate symptoms. CMV has also been implicated in the pathogenesis of several other causes of abdominal pain in AIDS. These include cholangiopathy and pancreatitis. HIV cholangiopathy commonly presents with fever, right upper quadrant pain and obstructive liver function tests. Both Cryptosporidia and Microsporidia species can also produce a similar sclerosing cholangitis-like picture. In all cases, biliary tree involvement is associated with a worse overall outcome.

Hepatosplenomegaly is often found in HIV infection. It may reflect infiltration by tumors, hepatitis from viral causes (e.g. hepatitis B or C or CMV) or mycobacterial infection. Medication-related hepatic disease is common, and can vary from asymptomatic mild elevation of bilirubin (noted with the protease inhibitor, indinavir) to life-threatening hepatitis or hepatic steatosis with other (often antiretroviral) agents. Ultrasound and CT scanning are useful investigations which allow both visualization and biopsy of specific lesions. They can also detect any associated abdominal lymphadenopathy which may be significant in patients with progressive HIV disease.

The effects of viral hepatitis are an increasing problem. This is a reflection of routes of transmission similar to those for HIV, together with a more rapid progression in co-infected patients. Management is complex and, as the outlook for HIV patients improves with HAART, so more thought needs to be given to the care of end-stage liver disease with its accompanying complications of cirrhosis, portal hypertension, bleeding, encephalopathy and hepatocellular carcinoma.

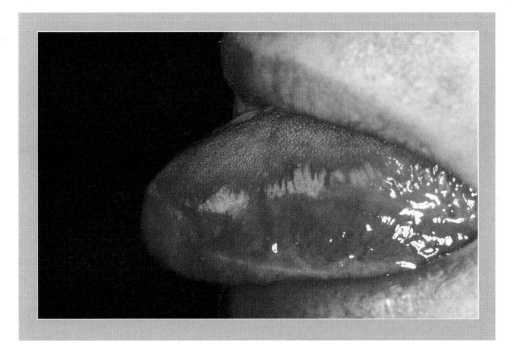

Figure 4.1   *Oral hairy leukoplakia* The whitish-gray corrugated lesions on the lateral margins of the tongue are characteristic of oral hairy leukoplakia (OHL). They are bilateral, and cannot be removed by scraping. Extensive OHL can spread onto the dorsal and ventral surfaces of the tongue. It can also be found on the buccal mucosa. OHL results from infection with Epstein–Barr virus which can be demonstrated in the lesions. Similar appearances may be seen in candidal leukoplakia, smoker's leukoplakia and epithelial dysplasia. If necessary, the diagnosis may be confirmed by biopsy. Like oral thrush, OHL indicates advancing HIV disease. Prior to the introduction of antiretrovirals and *Pneumocystis jiroveci* pneumonia prophylaxis, 75% of people with OHL progressed to AIDS within 3 years

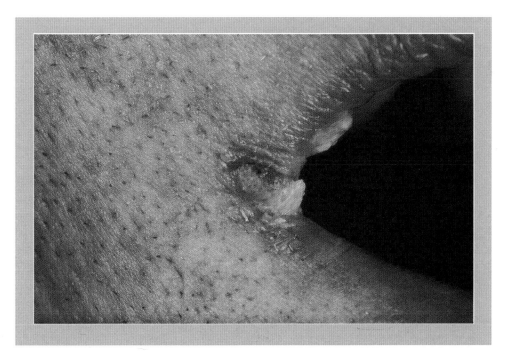

Figure 4.2   *Angular cheilitis* This condition is often associated with *Candida albicans* infection, although it can be seen by itself in advanced HIV disease

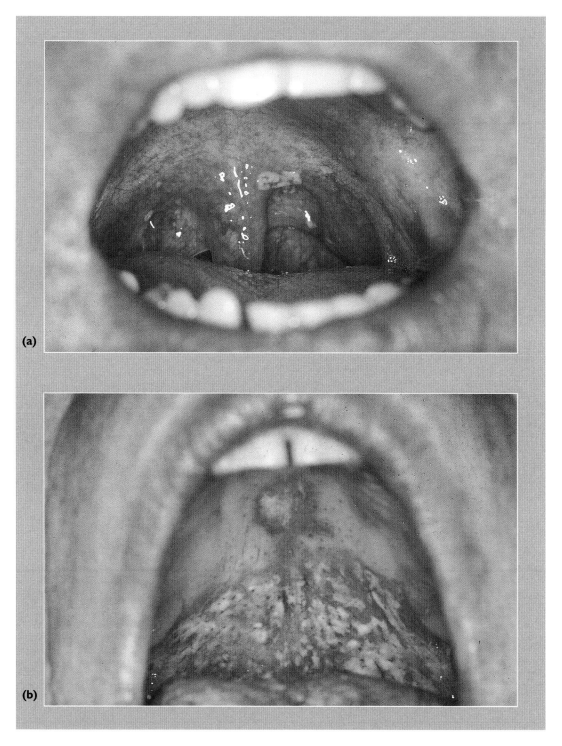

Figure 4.3   *Oral thrush* Thrush is due to *Candida albicans* in 95% of cases. It may present with loss of taste, a dry sore mouth or as a lesion reported by the patient. After an episode of HIV-related thrush there is 50% probability of developing a severe opportunistic infection in the next 2 years. HAART has reduced the reported incidence of candidiasis from over 30% to below 10%. This improvement in immunity directly correlates with increases in individual's blood CD4 counts. **(a and b)** Note the erythema as well as white plaques

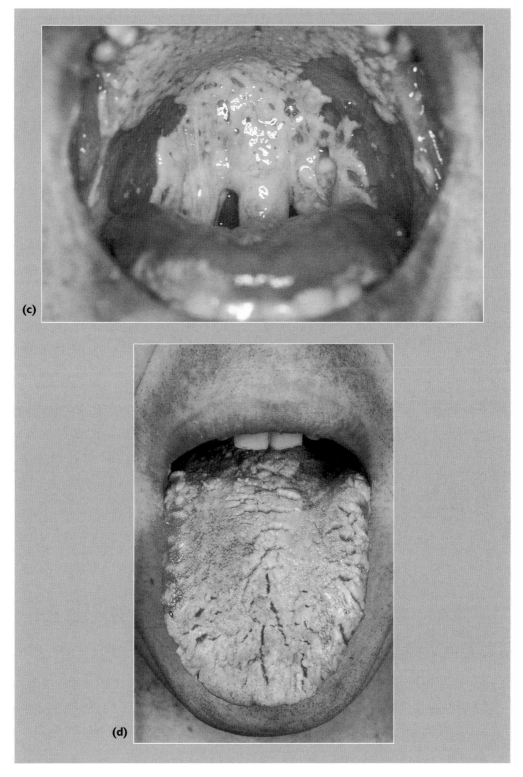

Figure 4.3 continued   Lack of response to standard therapy or extensive disease can result from concomitant antibiotic, cytotoxic or inhaled steroid administration. It can also indicate overgrowth by resistant organisms **(c)** and should be investigated by swabs for fungal culture and drug sensitivity.   Isolated lingual *Candida* **(d)** is rare and usually a furred tongue does not indicate disease

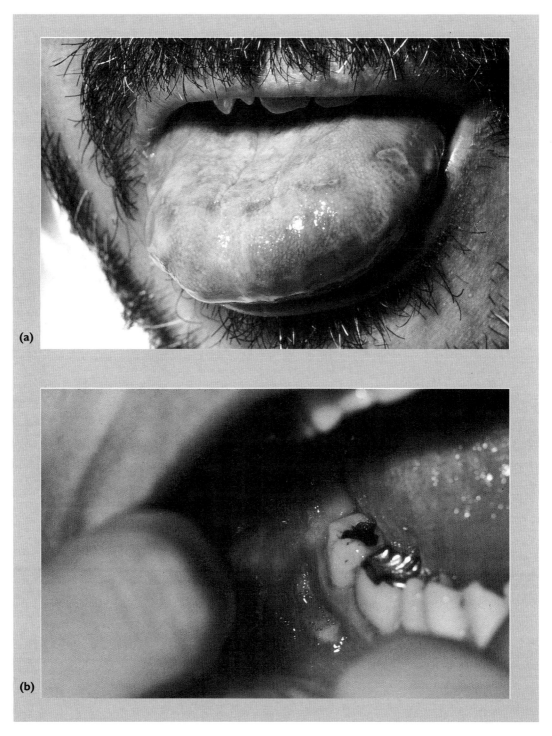

Figure 4.4 *Mouth ulceration* This usually presents with pain. It can be difficult to distinguish clinically between the different causes. **(a)** Note the swelling and ulceration due to herpes simplex infection (probably the most common cause). Oral ulceration due to CMV is rare although it can produce extensive disease with soft tissue necrosis. Aphthous ulceration may be minor (< 1 cm), major (> 1 cm) or herpetiform in appearance. It is usually found on non-keratinized epithelium and the lesion can be either solitary **(b)** or multiple. Histology of these ulcers reveals non-specific inflammation

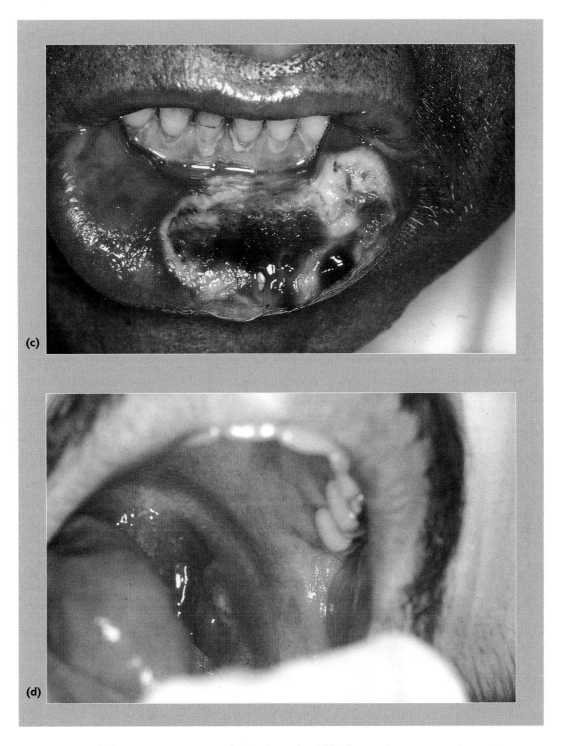

Figure 4.4 continued Culture-negative non-resolving ulcers should be biopsied since unusual organisms or tumors may present in this way, e.g. actinomycosis **(c)**. **(d)** A tonsillar B-cell tumor diagnosed on biopsy

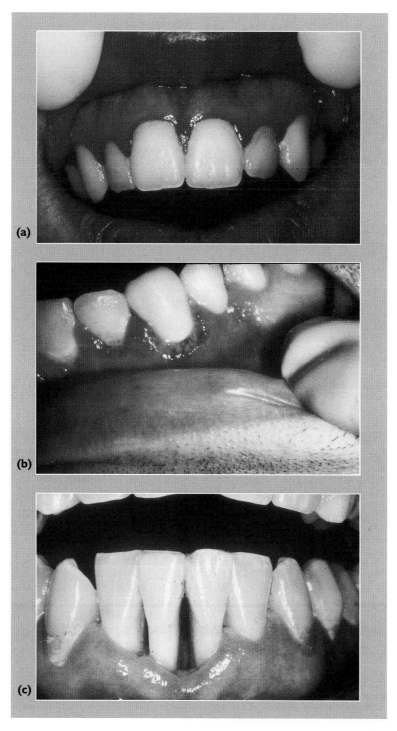

Figure 4.5   *Dental and gum disease* **(a)** *Linear gingival erythema* Advancing HIV infection is associated with increasing periodontal disease. This is reflected in biopsy samples as gingival infiltration by neutrophils, mast cells and macrophages. Clinically, this is most commonly seen as linear gingival erythema, formerly known as HIV gingivitis. Note the red band along the gingival margin which persisted after plaque removal and improved oral hygiene. The causative agent of this lesion remains to be defined, although some studies have implicated *Entamoeba gingivalis*. **(b)** *Necrotizing (ulcerative) gingivitis* There is destruction of the interdental papillae with resultant ulceration and sloughing. The patient complained of painful bleeding gums and bad breath. The lesion responded to antimicrobial therapy and cleaning. **(c)** *Necrotizing (ulcerative) peri-odontitis* Ulceration and necrosis has led to marked loss of both bone and soft tissue. The ulceration can recur and also extend across the mucogingival junction producing large areas of exposed underlying bone in the oral cavity. Cultures and histology of these lesions often fail to demonstrate a specific etiology, although secondary infection is common

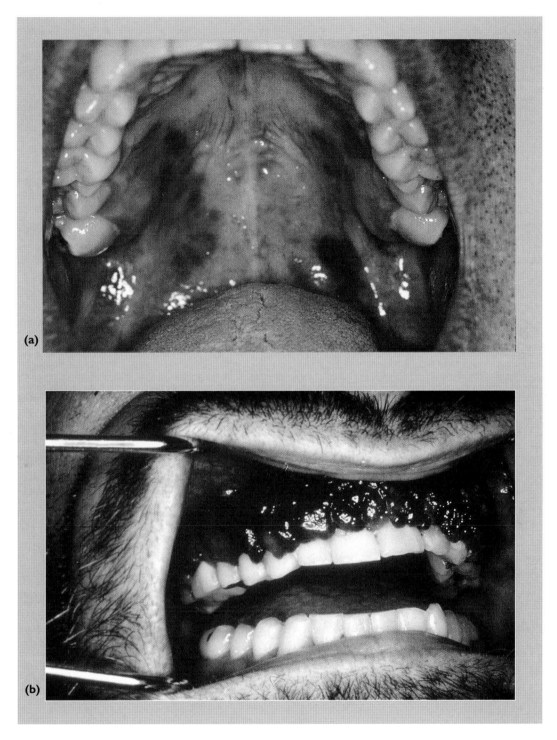

Figure 4.6 *Oral Kaposi's sarcoma* Kaposi's sarcoma usually involves the hard palate **(a)** and gingiva **(b)**, and presents as a red or purple flat or raised lesion in individuals with blood CD4 counts < 200 x 10^6/l. Unless it ulcerates and becomes infected, it will be painless. Extensive lesions, as demonstrated in Figure 8.11 in Chapter 8, may produce anorexia and weight loss through local physical effects. If a lesion grows rapidly or presents atypically then biopsy may be indicated to exclude other oral tumors such as lymphoma, or infections such as bacillary angiomatosis

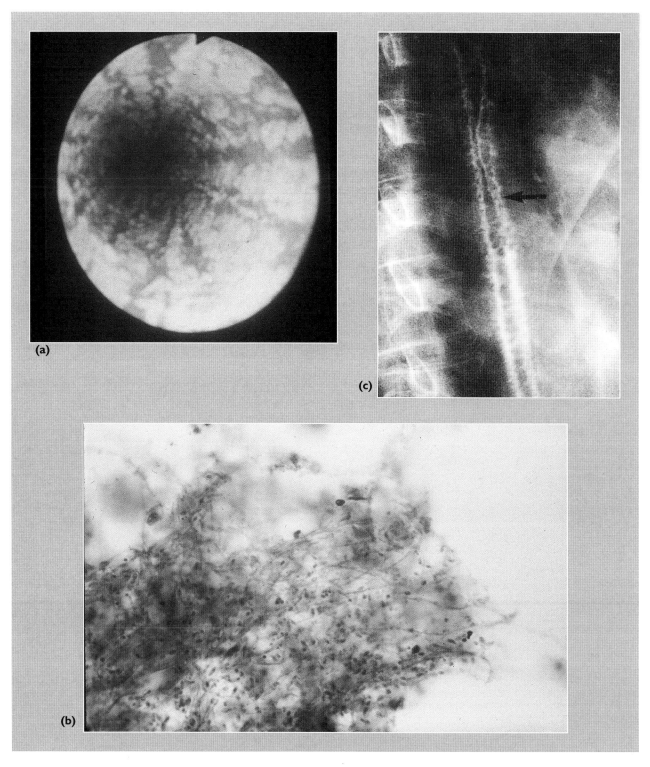

(a)

(c)

(b)

Figure 4.7 *Esophageal candida* Candida is responsible for 75% of all HIV-related esophageal symptoms. It can occur without obvious oral thrush being present. **(a)** An endoscopic view of the mid-esophagus showing extensive *Candida* almost entirely covering the mucosa that led to difficulty eating and marked weight loss. The candidal species had become resistant to standard antifungal therapy through long-term oral thrush prophylaxis. **(b)** *Candida pseudohyphae* and spores together with squamous cells in an esophageal brush specimen are seen. The barium swallow **(c)** shows fine mucosal ulceration and mamillation of the folds. The esophagus is small due to spasm. The patient complained of retrosternal discomfort on swallowing solid foods. He made a good response to systemic antifungal therapy. Barium swallows have largely been superseded by endoscopy for the diagnosis of HIV-associated dysphagia

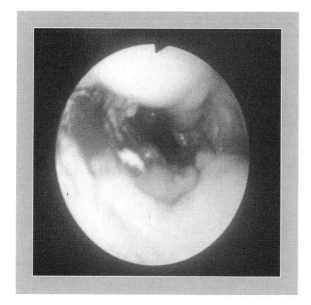

Figure 4.8 *Esophageal ulceration* Patients who have not responded to a trial of anti-candidal therapy are likely to have either CMV disease (up to 40%) or aphthous ulceration (30% of cases). The endoscopic view of the mid-esophagus shows extensive ulceration with ulcer slough. A more typical site for CMV disease is the lower esophagus

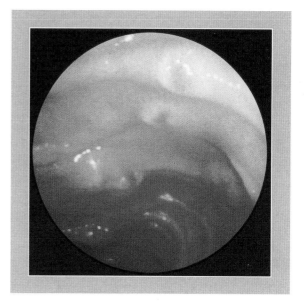

Figure 4.10 *Gastrointestinal lymphoma* An endoscopic view of the duodenum showing discrete mucosal ulcers. Biopsy revealed non-Hodgkin's B-cell lymphoma. HIV-related gastrointestinal lymphomas are often multicentric

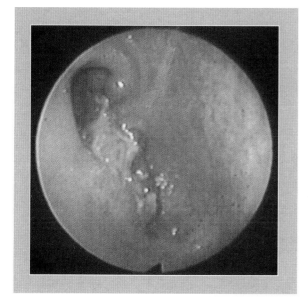

Figure 4.9 *Duodenal ulceration* An endoscopic view of the first part of the duodenum shows a punched out ulcer. The patient, with a CD4 count of $60 \times 10^6/l$, presented with a history of long-standing abdominal pain relieved by food. Biopsies revealed CMV 'owl's eye' inclusions with a marked inflammatory response. The pain and ulcer resolved with anti-CMV therapy. A clue to the diagnosis was that the patient had become persistently CMV PCR-positive in blood. This is a strong predictor of developing end-organ CMV disease, if no action is taken

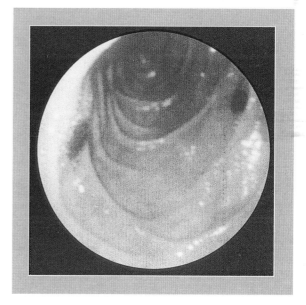

Figure 4.11 *Gastrointestinal Kaposi's sarcoma* An endoscopic view of the duodenum shows the raised purple lesions characteristic of Kaposi's sarcoma in a patient with extensive cutaneous disease complaining of abdominal pain and weight loss. Gastrointestinal Kaposi's sarcoma is found in up to 30% of patients with widespread skin or lymph node disease. Kaposi's sarcoma may infiltrate submucosally or ulcerate and bleed

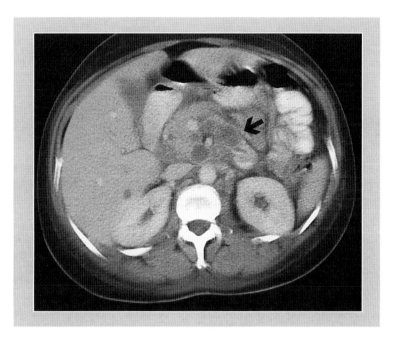

Figure 4.12   *Paraortic lymphadenopathy* The abdominal CT scan shows multiple low-density soft tissue masses at the origin of the superior mesenteric vessels (arrow). There is ring enhancement within the lymph nodes, which have displaced the pancreas anteriorly. Percutaneous needle biopsy revealed poorly formed granulomas with associated caseation. The sample was tuberculosis nucleic acid amplification (PCR) positive. The patient had presented with abdominal pain, night sweats, fevers and weight loss. The differential diagnosis of abdominal lymphadenopathy includes lymphoma, malignancy, mycobacterial and fungal disease. Although the ring enhancement suggests mycobacterial infection, tissue is needed to distinguish between the causes of lymphadenopathy. This can be obtained either as described in this case or, if necessary, surgically, using laparoscopic biopsy. The latter also enables peritoneal samples to be obtained for histology and culture

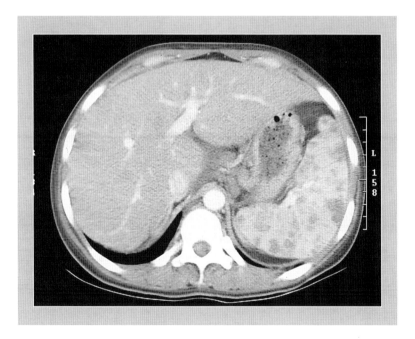

Figure 4.13   *Splenic abscesses* Abdominal disease is often part of a disseminated process. Physical examination may reveal lymphadenopathy at other sites which may be more amenable to biopsy. Multiple low-density splenic lesions in an African woman who presented with headache, fevers and hepatosplenomegaly are shown. She was noted to have large non-tender inguinal lymph nodes. Biopsy of these confirmed the clinical suspicion of mycobacterial disease. Massive splenomegaly is also a characteristic feature of visceral leishmaniasis. This should be considered in individuals who have spent any time in endemic areas

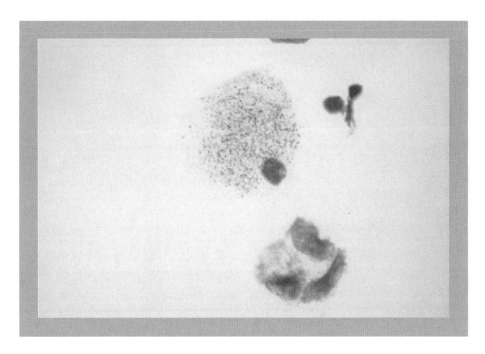

Figure 4.14   *Fine-needle aspiration* A fine-needle aspiration is shown of a lymph node containing mycobacterial organisms (staining red) engulfed within a macrophage. The large number of bacteria suggests atypical mycobacterial infection

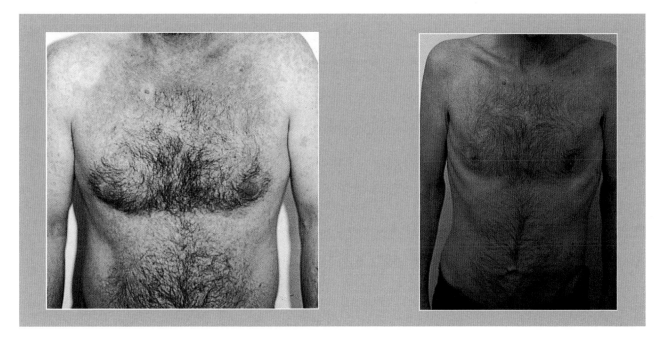

Figure 4.15   *Wasting* Many patients with advancing HIV infection lose weight. The illustrations show profound wasting in an AIDS patient over a 5-month period. This degree of weight loss is usually due to intercurrent infection or HIV wasting syndrome and presents predominantly as a loss of lean tissue mass. Diarrheal diseases are traditionally associated with weight loss, although in fact most severe opportunistic disease will cause wasting. If weight loss is due to poor nutrition or malabsorption (e.g. secondary to diarrhea) then useful weight gain may occur with hyperalimentation (using either parenteral or, if possible, enteral elemental diets). However, if an intercurrent infection is present but not treated, then the patient will continue to lose weight. Wasting is not only prognostically important but also has a considerable psychological impact on the individual. Recent work suggests that wasting can be reversed with HAART. Furthermore, the poor prognosis typically associated with this condition is greatly improved

Step	Sample	Investigation
1	stools and stools chart (at least three divided samples on consecutive days – best results with semiformed/liquid stool)	microscopy, culture for dysenteric pathogens, ova, cysts, parasites, mycobacterial culture, *Clostridium difficile* toxin (drug-induced pseudomembranous colitis), viral culture (CMV, herpes simplex virus, adenovirus)
	blood culture if febrile + mycobacterial culture if CD4 count < 100 x 10⁶/l	
2	flexible sigmoidoscopy and rectal biopsy	histology, bacteriology, mycobacteriology, virology
3	consider short course of metronidazole	
4	colonoscopy and biopsy ± ileoscopy	histology, bacteriology, mycobacteriology, virology
5	duodenoscopy and jejunoscopy – duodenal and jejunal brushing and biopsy	'HIV villous atrophy', ova, cysts, parasites, biopsy of macroscopic lesions
6	electron microscopy of tissue samples	Microsporidia species

Figure 4.16 *Stepwise investigation of HIV-related diarrhea* Many HIV-infected individuals will complain of occasional episodes of diarrhea. However, severe acute (seven loose stools for > 3 days) or chronic diarrhea (more than three loose stools per day, total weight > 200 g, for 1 month) should be investigated with the proposed guidelines. In general, pathogen detection is maximal in patients with weight loss and low CD4 counts (< 100 x 10⁶/l). At all steps of the algorithm, repeat stool samples are important, and improvements in staining techniques now allow almost all pathogens (including Microsporidia) to be diagnosed in this way. Three stool samples will lead to pathogen detection in 40% of patients, provided that appropriate tests are used, e.g. modified Ziehl–Neelsen for cryptosporidiosis and modified trichrome or Calcofluor stains for Microsporidia. The pick-up is not greatly increased by further samples, although this depends on availability of other investigations and on the laboratory support available.

Colonoscopy will detect isolated right-sided CMV disease which would have been missed using flexible sigmoidoscopy (present in 10–40% of cases where stool samples are negative but a pathogen is finally isolated). Colonoscopy allows ileoscopy to be performed. This increases the yield and may avert the need for upper gastrointestinal procedures. There is some evidence that jejunoscopy will detect more disease than duodenoscopy. This is largely due to an increased diagnosis of Microsporidia. Small bowel aspirates appear to add little to the overall strategy and are not recommended.

Electron microscopy will aid in the detection of pathogens that may not be seen easily using light microscopy, e.g. Microsporidia. It also enables speciation of this protozoon to be performed. However, it may not be cost-effective in many centers.

There are few definitive treatments for many of the opportunistic enteropathogens, and therefore HAART combined with symptomatic measures is often the best therapeutic strategy if the investigations do not yield a rapid result – especially in patients with higher CD4 counts (> 100 x 10⁶/l) and minimal systemic upset. As suggested in step 3 of the guidelines a short course of metronidazole may be a pragmatic approach while awaiting further investigations. If a patient is acutely unwell with diarrhea and fevers, then a quinolone antibiotic should be effective against possible bacterial causes

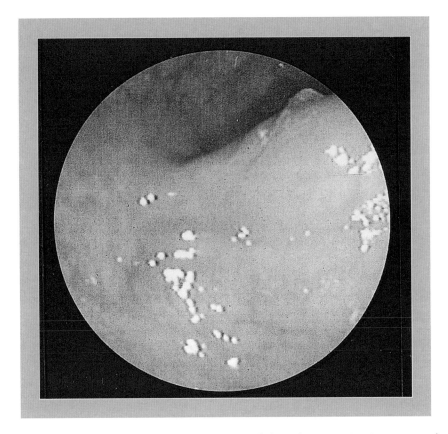

Figure 4.17   *The colon in chronic diarrhea* An endoscopic view of the colon in an AIDS patient with chronic pathogen-negative diarrhea. There is patchy mucosal edema with loss of the normal vascular pattern (which can be seen in an unaffected area in the background).   HIV has been demonstrated within the gastrointestinal epithelium in both the small and large bowel. Furthermore, the immune response within the gut mucosa is abnormal in both early and advanced HIV disease. Whether HIV is directly responsible for malabsorption (through 'villous atrophy' and impaired gut permeability) or diarrhea, however, remains unclear, as similar, although less marked, features are found in asymptomatic HIV infection. HAART will improve most cases of chronic diarrhea. This is more likely when a specific pathogen has been detected. Antiretroviral agents themselves can cause diarrhea, e.g. protease inhibitors, such as nelfinavir and ritonavir, although, in general, this is easily managed with symptomatic treatment. The return of chronic diarrhea usually implies a failure of the patient's HAART regimen

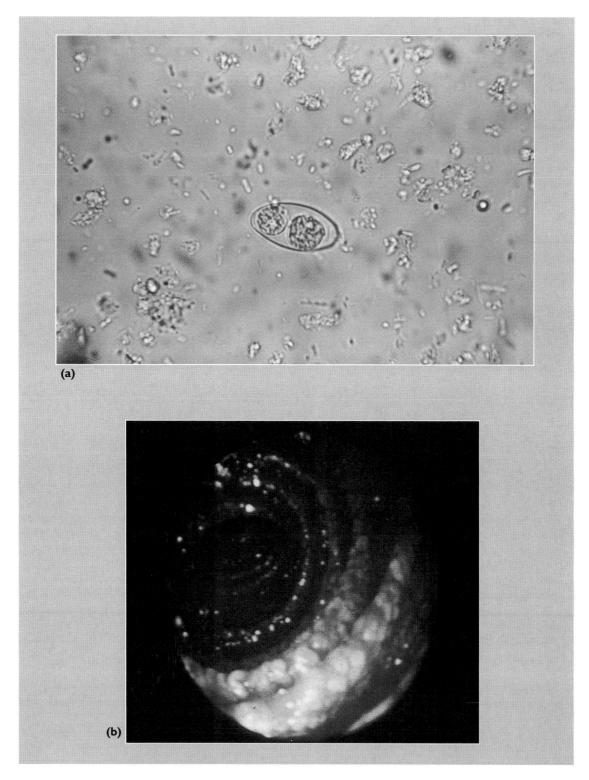

Figure 4.18   *Diarrhea – protozoa and bacteria* Asymptomatic carriage of amoebae **(a)** and *Giardia* is frequently seen in homosexual men.   Symptomatic infection is no more frequent in HIV-positive individuals, although can be more prolonged. Protozoan infection due to Cryptosporidium, *Isospora* and Microsporidia species are, however, common in HIV. Cryptosporidium is responsible for about 15% of all diarrhea in North American AIDS patients and up to 50% of AIDS-related diarrhea in Africa. It is acquired by drinking infected water. Recent work suggests that transmission is reduced if patients use only bottled water. Although boiling water should kill the oocyst, there is little evidence to support this practice. Water filters are of no benefit. **(b)** The edematous mucosal appearance of either severe cryptosporidiosis or microsporidiosis is shown

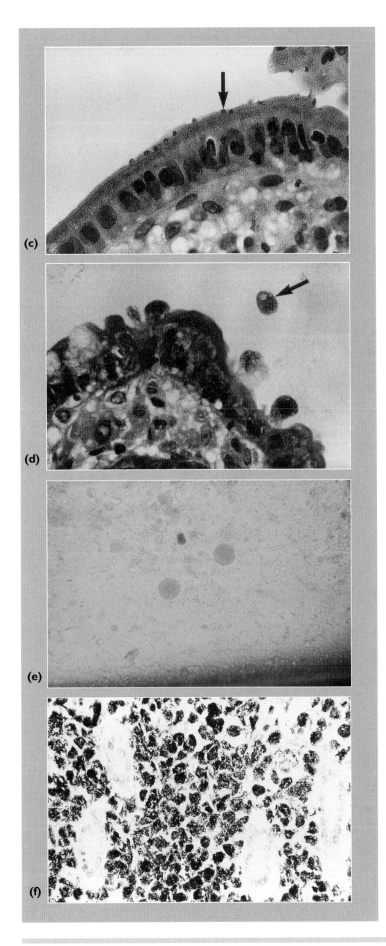

Figure 4.18 continued (c) Cryptosporidial organisms inhabit the brush border of the intestinal mucosa and can often be found throughout the gastrointestinal tract. A similar clinical picture of profuse watery diarrhea and varying abdominal pain is seen with Microsporidia species (**d**, staining black within the sloughed off enterocytes) and *Isospora belli* **(e)**. Microsporidial species (in particular *Enterocytozoon bieneusi*, as well as *Encepahalitozoon intestinalis* – which can also cause systemic disease) are now recognized as major HIV enteropathogens. Typically, these organisms are seen in late HIV disease (CD4 $< 150 \times 10^6$/l). Given the difficulty in diagnosing some protozoa with light microscopy, work has been directed at methods of DNA detection. These are not widely available but have a level of sensitivity approximately 1000 times greater than current techniques. HIV-infected patients have a high incidence of acute bacterial intestinal infection. For example, *Salmonella typhimurium* is 100 times more common and is often associated with bacteremia or recurrence. Mycobacterial diarrhea presents as a chronic illness with marked systemic features. Diagnosis is made by stool culture or biopsy. Inflammatory aggregates may be visible at endoscopy. **(f)** Abundant *Mycobacterium avium intracellulare complex* (MAC) are seen within a biopsy (ZN stain)

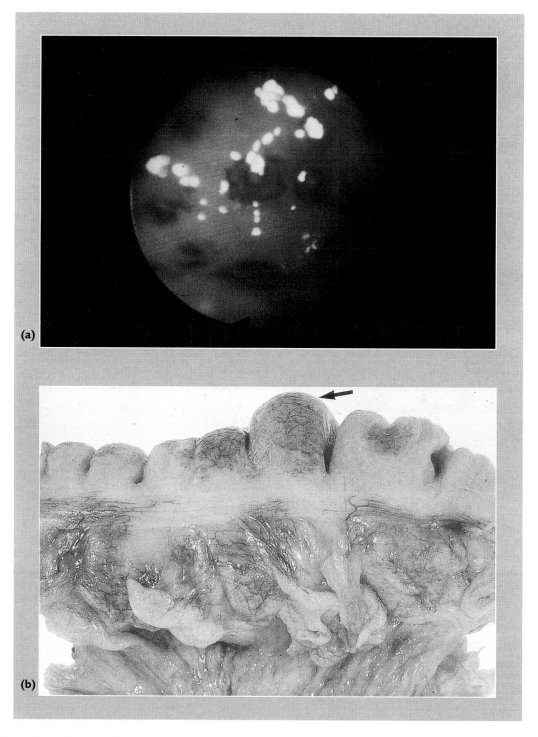

Figure 4.19   *Diarrhea – viral* CMV is the most common viral diarrheal pathogen (20% of cases). It can cause a wide variety of enteral diseases, although it usually presents as colitis. Its sigmoidoscopic appearance is non-specific and may range from hyperemia to hemorrhage and ulceration **(a)**. CMV colitis may be severe and progress to ileocecal obstruction, toxic megacolon, ischemic necrosis and perforation. **(b)** Inflamed 'diverticulitis' in the colon which resulted from destruction of the muscularis layer is shown

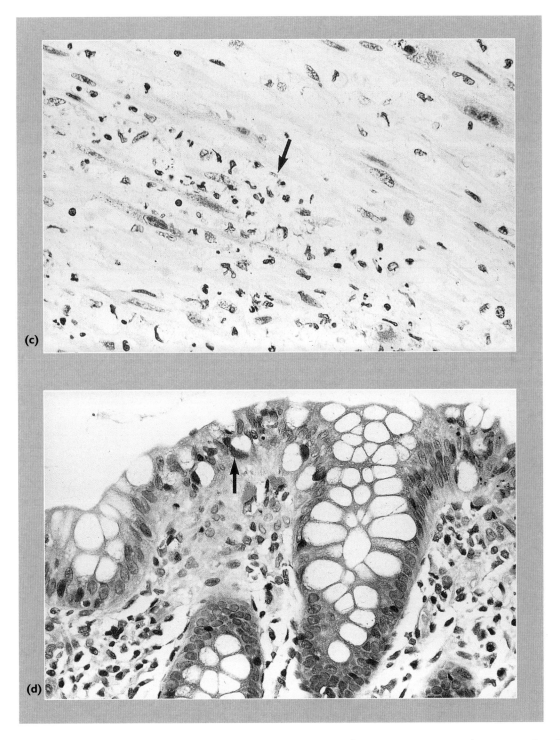

Figure 4.19 continued **(c)** This is seen in detail here, where an intense inflammatory response is demonstrated within the circular muscular layer of the colon. Adenovirus-associated diarrhea has recently been documented in AIDS patients. Unlike CMV, it tends to produce chronic watery diarrhea. This results from superficial mucosal infection, sparing deeper structures. **(d)** Basophilic adenovirus inclusions are seen within the nuclei of endothelial cells (smudge cells). It can be easily missed and may be more common than its estimated prevalence of 5%. Herpes simplex can cause diarrhea and distal colitis. Here, bowel disease is usually associated with obvious skin and perianal involvement

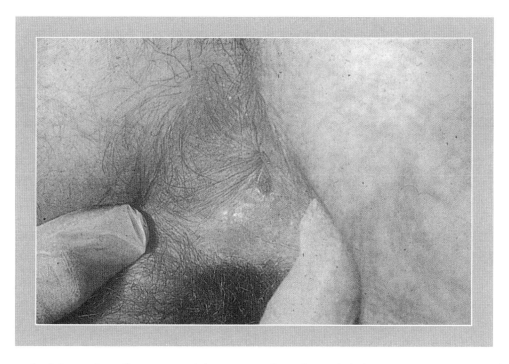

Figure 4.20 *Anal chancre* Sexually transmitted disease must always be excluded in patients presenting with genital and anal lesions. The perianal ulceration shown was due to syphilis

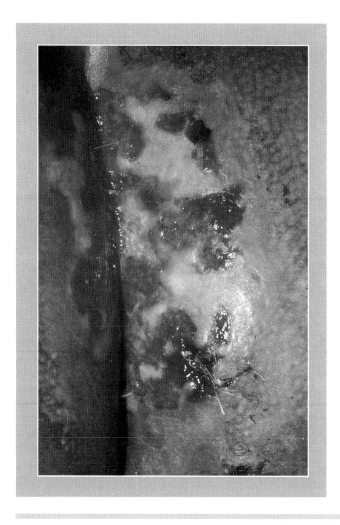

Figure 4.21 *Perianal herpes* Severe ulceration and edema affecting the perianal area is seen in a man with profound immunosuppression and a history of recurrent herpetic disease. The lesions had not responded to antiherpes therapy and biopsy demonstrated aciclovir-resistant herpes. This should be considered in patients presenting with extensive disease and low CD4 counts ($< 100 \times 10^6/l$)

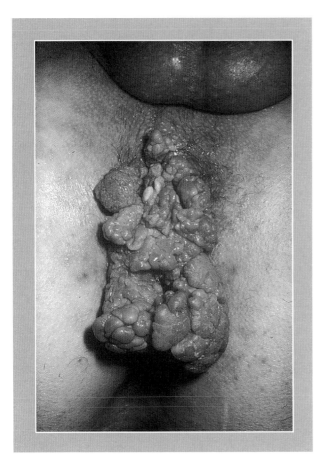

Figure 4.22 *Perianal warts* There are florid exophytic warts almost completely obscuring the anus. This extensive disease is a feature of late HIV infection and is often difficult to treat. Human papilloma virus (HPV), predominantly type 16, is associated with anal intraepithelial neoplasia (AIN). HIV-infected individuals are at increased risk of harboring these strains, and AIN is one of the most common non-AIDS-defining illnesses among homosexual men. Therefore, patients with chronic genital warts should be monitored with regular cytological examination. Recent evidence suggests that there is a high prevalence of HPV in HIV-infected individuals whether or not they have had anal sex. This translates into an increased risk of AIN. Some authorities suggest that all individuals with blood CD4 counts < 500 x 10^6/l should be offered regular anal cytological screening

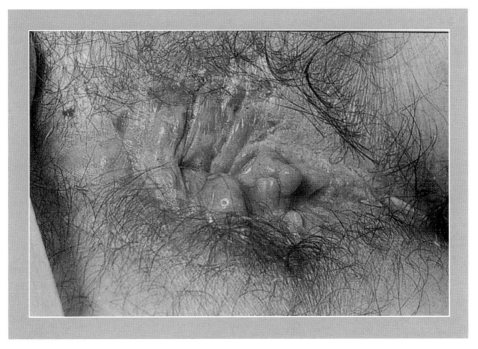

Figure 4.23 *Chronic perianal disease* There is superficial ulceration, fissuring, warts and skin tags. The edematous appearance resulted from acute on chronic infection. The patient complained of pain and tenesmus. Swabs from the ulcers grew herpes, and the pain settled with aciclovir, local anesthetics and stool softeners. Chronic perianal disease often requires a surgical examination, although most management is conservative. Anal herpes may present as a long-standing fissure. Extensive disease involving the anal sphincter (especially due to CMV) can lead to progressive fecal incontinence

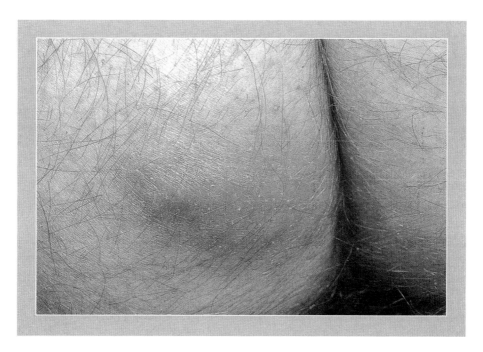

Figure 4.24 *Perianal abscess* The large abscess is starting to point but required formal incision and drainage. Two weeks later the patient was examined under anesthesia which revealed a fistula-*in-ano*

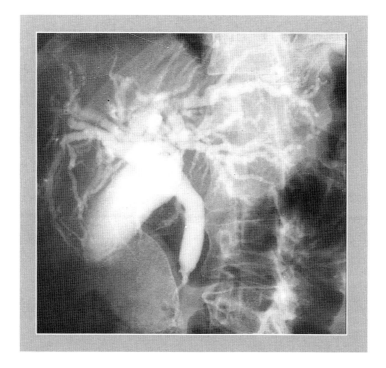

Figure 4.25 *HIV cholangiopathy* The radiograph taken during endoscopic retrograde cholangiopancreatography resembles sclerosing cholangitis. There are multiple stenoses and dilatations in the intrahepatic ducts. Note also the stricture at the lower end of the common bile duct and the dilated gall bladder. The clinical picture is similar to that of acalculous cholecystitis which can be readily diagnosed on ultrasound and is also found in advanced disease. Both conditions present with fever, abdominal pain and right upper quadrant tenderness. Jaundice is a late event but, in HIV cholangiopathy, the alkaline phosphatase will be increased up to 20 times the upper limit of normal. A wide variety of pathogens have been implicated in both conditions. These include Cryptosporidia, Microsporidia, CMV, *Mycobacterium avium complex*, Kaposi's sarcoma and lymphoma. Patients with both pathogen-positive diarrhea and HIV cholangiopathy obtain less benefit on HAART than patients with diarrhea alone. This applies to both symptom and pathogen control

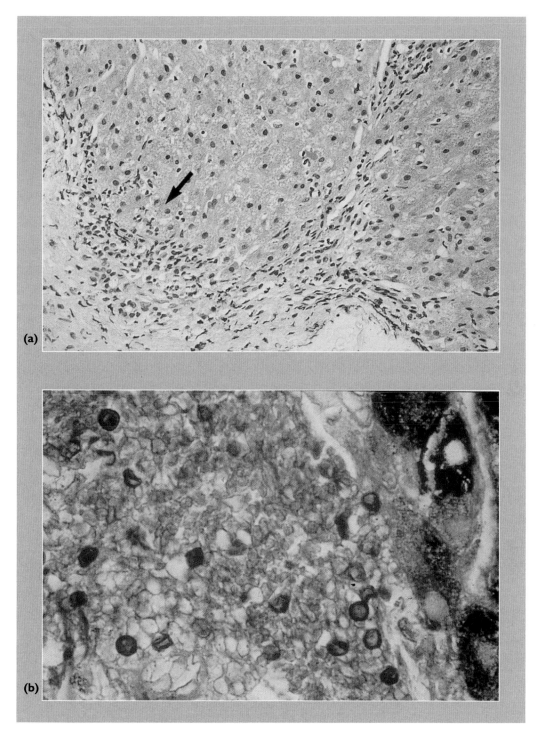

Figure 4.26 *Liver disease* The modes of transmission of HIV infection are the same as those of many hepatitis viruses. HIV-related immunosuppression can profoundly alter the clinical picture of these viruses. In some cases (e.g. hepatitis B), the disease seems to be milder if HIV is also present. Conversely, hepatitis C (predominantly transmitted through blood) is a more aggressive disease with HIV co-infection. The liver biopsy from a case of hepatitis C **(a)** shows lobular and portal inflammation and apoptotic hepatocytes. This is reflected in persistently deranged liver function tests. Opportunistic hepatic pathogens are common, and often tissue is required to establish the nature of the disease. Liver function tests can provide some clues to the etiology. For example, jaundice suggests sepsis or cholangitis and a raised alkaline phosphatase suggests inflammation (*Mycobacterium avium complex* or CMV) or neoplastic infiltration. The main indications for liver biopsy (after ultrasound imaging) are pyrexias of unknown origin, hepatomegaly or persistently abnormal liver function tests. **(b)** Scattered cysts of *Pneumocystis* are demonstrated within an expanded sinusoid in an AIDS patient who presented with hepatomegaly and a small pleural effusion

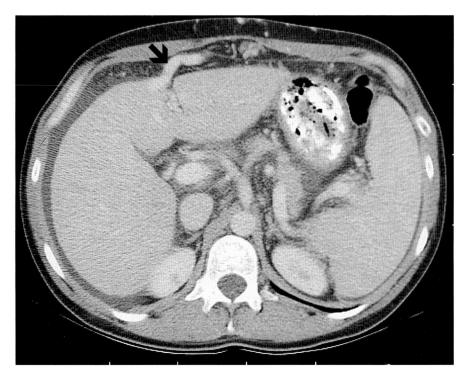

Figure 4.27 *Portal hypertension from liver cirrhosis* With increased survival from HAART and improved treatment of opportunistic infections, there is now a greater number of patients with chronic co-infections such as hepatitis B and C. All HIV-infected patients should be tested for hepatitis A, B and C infection. If negative on screening, they should be re-tested on a regular basis. The portal phase of a liver CT scan is shown. The features of portal hypertension are present: the para-umbilical vein, coming off the left portal vein, is recanalized (arrow). Ascites is present around the liver, which itself shows minor surface irregularity, consistent with established cirrhosis.

The patient's hepatitis B infection may be mild in untreated HIV since hepatic damage depends on a functioning host immune response. However, there can be very high levels of hepatitis B viral replication, leading to fibrosing cholestatic hepatitis. Hepatitis B may reactivate in advanced HIV disease, although clearing of hepatitis B on HAART has been reported. Immune recovery disease may worsen symptoms of underlying infection. As HAART drugs can be hepatotoxic, there may be diagnostic confusion when there is derangement of liver function tests after commencing a new regimen. Immune recovery disease causing flare of hepatitis B has been reported and can be severe. This can also follow withdrawal of treatment such as lamivudine

Hepatitis B and HIV

Assessment	Investigations
Full clinical assessment including alcohol consumption, history of jaundice, injecting drug use, psychiatric disease, physical examination	HBV sAg, HBeAg, anti-HAV IgG, full blood count, clotting, liver ultrasound
Advice on alcohol consumption, risk and routes of transmission, complications and treatment options	liver biopsy to stage disease, if not clinically contraindicated. Disease may be classified as mild, moderate or severe on the basis of a modified Ishak necroinflammatory score
	immunize against HAV if not already immune; may not respond

HBV, hepatitis B virus; HBeAg, hepatitis B e antigen; HAV, hepatitis A virus; IgG, immunoglobulin G

Treatment

The available treatment options are at present interferon-α (IFN-α), 3TC (lamivudine), adefovir and tenofovir. At present, it is only possible to obtain them through trials or on compassionate release. IFN-α has a very low response rate in HIV infection. 3TC monotherapy may lead to HBV- and HIV-drug resistance.

Mild disease Unlikely to respond to IFN-α. HIV therapy alone may clear infection. If 3TC is part of treatment regimen, withdrawal may cause a flare of HBV.

Moderate disease Where CD4 counts are high, IFN-α has been effective, but treatment is not easily tolerated. 3TC will inhibit HBV viral replication and can be used if clinically indicated. If 3TC is withdrawn it may cause a flare of clinical disease. The situation should be carefully discussed with the patient who may elect to await better treatment options. Optimizing HAART may clear HBV infection.

Cirrhosis Consider β-blockade if portal hypertension. Consider transplant if HIV progonosis good. In advanced disease, 3TC may cause clinical improvement, but if transplant is considered this should be discussed with regional transplant unit in advance.

Figure 4.28   Investigation and management of hepatitis B

Hepatitis C and HIV

Assessment	Investigations
Initial assessment is much as for hepatitis B, outlined in Figure 4.28	HCV antibody. There may be false-negatives among patients with HIV; it may be necessary to perform PCR-based viral load on patients with persistently elevated liver function tests
	HBSAg, anti-HBS and anti-HAV IgG
	full blood count and clotting studies
	liver function tests and ultrasound
	consider liver biopsy where clinically appropriate. Liver damage is assessed as for hepatitis B by modified Ishak score
	HCV genotype if treatment contemplated

Hepatitis C virus (HCV) disease is more common among HIV-infected individuals, especially among injecting drug users and hemophiliacs (60–90%). There is some evidence of sexual transmission of the virus; non-injecting partners of injecting drug users have a higher prevalence of infection, as do children of infected mothers. Acute hepatitis C infection is increasingly recognized among non-injecting HIV-infected individuals – this may manifest as an asymptomatic transaminitis of unknown cause.

HCV may progress more rapidly in HIV-infected individuals; rises in blood CD4 counts may be impaired in the co-infected. Whereas in the immunocompetent, 20–30% will progress to cirrhosis within 15–30 years, a higher proportion of patients with HIV will progress and at a faster rate. Viremia may be higher and is inversely correlated with CD4 count. Alcohol use, HBV infection and age are all adverse prognosticators. HCV genotype also affects prognosis – type 1, the most common genotype, may be less responsive to treatment which may need to be prolonged. Many antiretrovirals may be hepatotoxic; this may be more severe in HCV-infected individuals. HAART does not appear to affect the rate of cirrhosis.

Treatment

All patients with HIV/HCV co-infection should be assessed at least once for possible treatment. Patients with well-preserved CD4 counts may respond as well as HIV-negative individuals. Criteria for treatment are therefore the same in HIV-positive and -negative individuals. Decision to treat is based on the status of HCV and HIV; HCV is usually treated first if the HIV disease is stable.

Management of patients should be performed in a specialist unit with close liaison with local hepatology and liver transplant services. Patients with incipient or established cirrhosis should be assessed with liver ultrasound and α-fetoprotein on a regular basis as there is a 3–4% annual risk of developing hepatocellular carcinoma.

The current standard of care for immunocompetent individuals is interferon/ribavirin. Sustained response rates in this group are in the region of 50%, although this may vary with genotype. Newer formulations such as pegylated interferons have been shown to be more effective than standard interferons.

Side-effects of treatment may be severe and include flu-like symptoms, anemia, cytopenias and depression. There is a theoretical risk of interaction between ribavirin and certain antiretroviral drugs such as zidovudine and stavudine, although this has not been confirmed in clinical practice. There is no reason for HIV-positive patients to be denied interferon/ribavirin treatment even if on HAART. All patients should be considered for HAV and HBV vaccination if not already immune.

Mild disease Patients may elect to defer treatment, in which case they should be kept under regular review with repeat liver biopsy in 2–3 years.

Moderate-severe disease Consider treatment: 6–12 months of interferon/ribavirin or pegylated interferon/ribavirin. There are limited data on co-infected individuals as yet.

Severe disease In established cirrhosis, patients may be candidates for transplantation where HIV is well controlled. Interferon is contraindicated in hepatic decompensation. In compensated disease, it may be given in reduced dose with frequent monitoring.

Figure 4.29   Investigation and management of hepatitis C

5

Endocrine, metabolic, musculoskeletal and renal disease

ADRENAL INSUFFICIENCY

The hypothalamic–pituitary–adrenal axis is frequently subclinically deranged in HIV disease, although frank, clinically evident adrenal insufficiency is uncommon and usually occurs only in advanced infection. There is often slight basal serum hypercortisolemia with lower dehydroepiandrosterone (DHEA) concentrations; these generally do not require treatment. This high ratio of cortisol : DHEA levels may induce a worsening in immune status by shifting the cytokine production from the so-called TH1 or cellular-type response (interferon-α, IL-2 and IL-12) to the TH2 or humoral-type response (IL-4, IL-5, IL-6 and IL-10), a hallmark of HIV-disease progression.

Clinical adrenal insufficiency does not tend to occur until more than 80% of the gland has been destroyed. However, up to two-thirds of patients with AIDS may have adrenal involvement. The most common pathogen is CMV (detected at post-mortem in 50% of patients). In most cases, this virus rarely causes more than 60% adrenal necrosis.

Other causes of adrenal destruction include: infection – *Mycobacterium tuberculosis* and *Mycobacterium avium intracellulare* complex (MAC), *Cryptococcus neoformans*, *Histoplasma capsulatum*, *Pneumocystis jiroveci* and *Toxoplasma gondii*; neoplasms – Kaposi's sarcoma and lymphoma; hemorrhage, fibrosis and infarction. Adrenocortical antibodies are detected in a substantial proportion of HIV-infected individuals. Drugs may reduce steroidogenesis (ketoconazole), enhance cortisol metabolism (rifamycins), or suppress pituitary secretion of corticotropin due to their intrinsic glucocorticoid activity (megestrol acetate). Overt

Cushing's syndrome has been described with megestrol treatment.

Fatigue and postural hypotension are often seen late in HIV infection, although the contribution of adrenal insufficiency is probably small. A short synacthen test is useful for screening and further investigations are rarely needed. Impaired pituitary reserve is common (25% of symptomatic patients), although overt deficiency is rare. Should investigations suggest cortisol deficiency, it is prudent to perform a full screen of anterior pituitary function. Low cortisol concentrations should be treated irrespective of the etiology.

Basal aldosterone concentrations tend to be lower in HIV-infected individuals, and both hyporeninemic and hyper-reninemic hypoaldosteronism have been reported.

THYROID DISEASE

Clinically significant opportunistic infection of the thyroid is rare. The most common presentation is invasion by *Pneumocystis* leading to a neck mass and a transient period of hyperthyroidism, followed by reduced glandular function. Diagnosis can be made on needle aspiration. Outside these isolated cases, thyroid function tends to be normal in HIV infection.

HYPOGONADISM

Low serum testosterone has been reported in up to 40% of HIV-infected males and in 50% of patients with AIDS. As well as its association with advanced HIV infection, it is more common in injecting drug users and in patients with weight loss. It can affect both men and women. Complaints, possibly related to hypogonadism, are non-specific and include decreased libido, erectile dysfunction, gynecomastia and muscle wasting. In addition to a direct HIV effect, chronic hypercortisolemia may contribute to gonadal dysfunction and reduced androgen secretion. Children with HIV infection will commonly fail to thrive, have growth restriction and a delayed puberty. This is not just a reflection of malnutrition and probably results from impaired production of both gonadal and growth hormones. Testicular infection may occur from CMV, MAC, *Toxoplasma gondii* or tuberculosis. HIV DNA has been found in 5–20% of spermatogonia and spermatocytes. Drugs such as ketoconazole, heroin, alcohol and methadone may also suppress androgen production.

Testosterone concentrations may vary during the day, peaking in the early morning. Therefore, the time of the assay should be noted when measuring testosterone levels. The most useful laboratory indicator is serum free testosterone concentration. Follicle stimulating hormone (FSH) and luteinizing hormone (LH) as well as estradiol, should also be assessed, as evidence suggests that the majority of hypogonadism (80%) results from either a central (hypothalamic or pituitary) or mixed central and peripheral (testicular) defect.

The efficacy and safety of testosterone therapy in HIV infection is debatable. Administration of treatment doses of testosterone to HIV-infected men may result in improved quality of life. Some, but not all, studies have shown increases in weight, lean body mass and muscle strength. The downside is a possible increase in hormone-dependent tumors and avascular necrosis.

HYPERLIPIDEMIA

Elevated triglycerides and low-density lipoprotein (LDL) are common among patients taking protease inhibitors (PIs). Figure 5.1 shows a centrifuged blood sample from a patient with grossly elevated lipid levels. Up to 75% of patients taking PIs have high lipids (typically, raised triglycerides with or without increases in cholesterol, such as Figure 5.1), and may be at risk of long-term heart disease. However, HIV

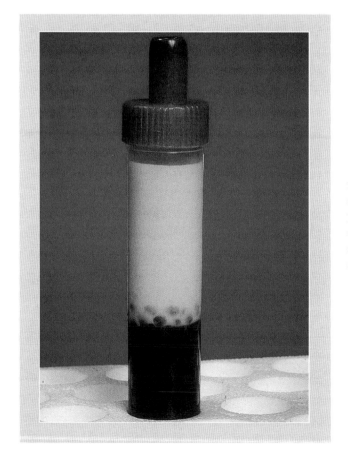

Figure 5.1 *Hyperlipidemia* A centrifuged blood sample from a patient with grossly elevated lipid levels. The milky serum represents very low-density lipoprotein (VLDL) particles which contain triglyceride and cholesterol, and remain in suspension. It should be noted that an elevation in the LDL-cholesterol fraction alone will result in a clear serum sample

itself is a recognized cause of lipid abnormalities, generally promoting a decline in high-density lipoprotein (HDL) and an increase in triglyceride levels. Isolated cholesterol abnormalities occur in patients taking regimens that do not include PIs. This includes both nucleoside and non-nucleoside reverse transcriptase inhibitor (NNRTI)-based combinations. In the latter case, this is more often elevated total cholesterol, together with an increase in 'protective' levels of HDL. Raised concentration of homocysteine can also occur, which is associated with increased cardiovascular disease risk.

LIPODYSTROPHY

Fat redistribution associated with other metabolic abnormalities was described soon after the widespread release of protease inhibitors (PIs). Adipose redistribution can be divided as fat accumulation (lipohypertrophy), including truncal obesity, visceral fat deposition, breast hypertrophy and enlargement of the dorsocervical pad ('buffalo hump; Figure 5.2), and fat wasting (lipoatrophy). The latter is specifically seen in HIV infection and is often most apparent in the face and limbs. Central obesity is the

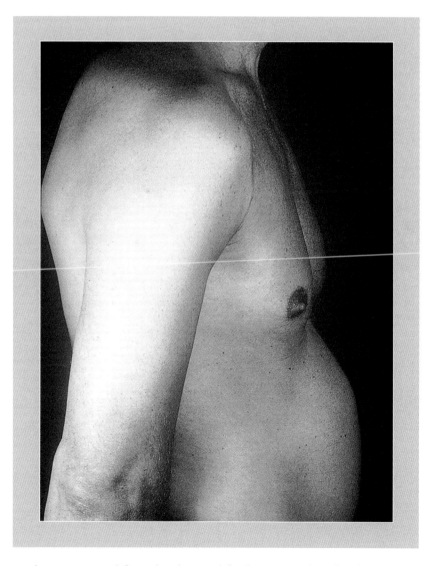

Figure 5.2 *Lipohypertrophy* Dorsocervical fat pad and visceral fat deposition. These lipodystrophic changes may be associated with hyperlipidemia, hyperinsulinemia and insulin resistance. The prevalence of fat redistribution is estimated at between 50 and 75% of all patients on HAART

Full case definition	Clinical and laboratory data (but no body imaging data)	Clinical data (but no body imaging or laboratory data)
Female gender	gender	age
Age over 40 years	age	HIV duration
HIV duration >4 years	HIV duration	CDC category
CDC category C	CDC category	CD4 change from nadir
Increased waist : hip ratio	waist : hip ratio	waist circumference
Decreased HDL cholesterol	estimated HDL cholesterol	
Increased anion gap	triglycerides	
Increased ratio of visceral adipose tissue to subcutaneous adipose tissue (> 1.59)	lactate anion gap	
Increased trunk to limb fat ratio		
Decreased leg fat percentage (< 8.8%)		

(a)

Fasting hyperlipidemia (total cholesterol > 5.5 mmol/l (> 220 mg/dl) or triglycerides > 2.0 mmol/l (> 170 mg/dl))

Elevated fasting glucose (6.1–7.0 mmol/l (109–126 mg/dl)) or diabetes mellitus (fasting glucose > 7.0 mmol/l (> 126 mg/dl))

Impaired 2-h glucose tolerance test

(b)

Figure 5.3 *Criteria for diagnosis of HAART-related lipodystrophy* Such criteria are not fully defined, although the above have been proposed. **(a)** This model used data drawn from 417 cases of (doctor and patient agreed) lipodystrophy compared to HIV-infected controls. The best model requires body composition measurements using DEXA or CT scans. Without these it is more applicable to routine clinical practice, although the sensitivity and specificity fall from 80% and 79%, respectively. The figures given under full case definition (e.g. age over 40 years) are values that will score most highly within the case definition (see www.ti3m.com/hiv/default_ld.htm). **(b)** Lipid abnormalities associated with HIV

most commonly reported feature (60%), followed by peripheral wasting (50%) and facial wasting (40%). They can occur with antiretrovirals other than PIs, e.g. nucleosides, such as stavudine, didanosine and lamivudine, or even in untreated HIV infection. However, the strongest association is with PIs. Other risk factors are duration of exposure to HAART, female sex and body mass index at the start of treatment.

The criteria for diagnosis of HAART-related lipodystrophy are given in Figure 5.3, together with the lipid abnormalities associated with HIV.

The mechanism of fat redistribution has not been clearly defined, and it may arise in a number of ways. These include drug-induced inhibition of several host-cell proteins involved in lipid and carbohydrate metabolism, PI-induced subcutaneous adipocyte apoptosis, mitochondrial toxicity from nucleoside-analogs and cytokine dysregulation in the setting of immune recovery.

Assessment of body fat changes can be either subjective (reported by patient, carer or health professional) or objective (DEXA scan for limb fat, cross-sectional CT or MR scan for visceral fat). The latter tests are most useful in detecting fat redistribution. They can be supplemented by bioelectrical impedance analysis, which may be helpful in monitoring wasting.

DIABETES

Frank diabetes following PI treatment has been described, but is not common. The incidence is reported as 4% after 1 year of PI treatment, with 8% showing impaired glucose tolerance. It is more frequent among patients who have a family history of diabetes, are older and are obese. There is a strong association between the presence of lipodystrophy and the development of diabetes. Insulin resistance has also been reported among patients taking nucleosides with PIs and non-nucleosides. Some of this is reversible, as insulin sensitivity often returns after PIs are discontinued.

MITOCHONDRIAL TOXICITY

Nucleoside analogs have been implicated in mitochondrial damage in the context of HIV, particularly with the NRTIs, stavudine and zidovudine. Their effect is believed to be mediated by incorporation into mitochondrial polymerase-γ. Syndromes associated with mitochondrial damage include pancreatitis, neurotoxicity, myopathy, lactic acidosis, bone marrow suppression and liver toxicity. Protease inhibitors may compound the effect.

ACUTE PANCREATITIS

Hyperamylasemia may arise from both pancreatic and salivary gland sources. Distinction can be made on the basis of differing electrophoretic mobility. Although this is not a standard investigation, it may be helpful when patients are noted to have elevated blood amylase on laboratory tests, and new abdominal symptoms. This is often seen in those with hepatitis B or C infection, or taking medication such as co-trimoxazole or didanosine. The most common causes of acute pancreatitis are alcohol excess and prescribed medication. The abdominal CT scan in Figure 5.4 shows acute pancreatitis resulting from intravenous pentamidine. Figure 5.5 is the abdominal CT scan of a heavy alcohol drinker who developed recurrent episodes of pancreatitis while on nebulized pentamidine. It shows chronic calcific pancreatic disease.

Grossly elevated triglyceride concentrations can also induce pancreatitis. This may be related to PI therapy but also occurs with NRTIs and in the presence of normal lipids. Opportunistic infections are a relatively infrequent cause of acute pancreatitis. CMV (5%) and MAC (2%) are the most common reported conditions.

LACTIC ACIDOSIS

Mitochondrial toxicity contributes to a range of disorders of lactate metabolism, from asymptomatic hyperlactatemia to frank and fatal type-B lactic acidosis. The NRTIs, stavudine, zidovudine, lamivudine, didanosine and abacavir have all been implicated, although PIs may also contribute. Symptoms in early acidosis are often non-specific, and include unexplained tiredness, nausea, abdominal pain, weight loss and dyspnea. It may progress rapidly to death. Treatment is at present empirical, but aggressive supportive measures including intensive-care monitoring may be required. Various treatments, including coenzyme Q, riboflavin and dichloroacetate, have been tried but none has been properly evaluated. At present, there is little evidence to suggest that blood lactate concentrations should be routinely measured in asymptomatic individuals on treatment. If they are requested for a clinical indication, blood should be rapidly transported to the laboratory or on ice to avoid spurious elevation. Severe symptoms are associated with blood lactate levels at least three times the upper limit of the normal range.

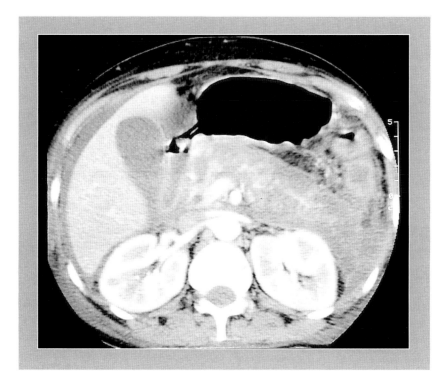

Figure 5.4 *Acute pancreatitis* Abdominal CT scan showing acute pancreatitis caused by intravenous pentamidine. This drug is responsible for up to 30% of cases, and has a direct toxic effect on pancreatic islet cells. Patients will have hypoglycemia followed by diabetes mellitus once most of the endocrine cells are damaged. The NRTI, didanosine, is another common cause of pancreatitis (10% of cases). The effect is dose-dependent and is more likely in individuals with a previous history of pancreatitis. In a small number of individuals the episode may be life-threatening

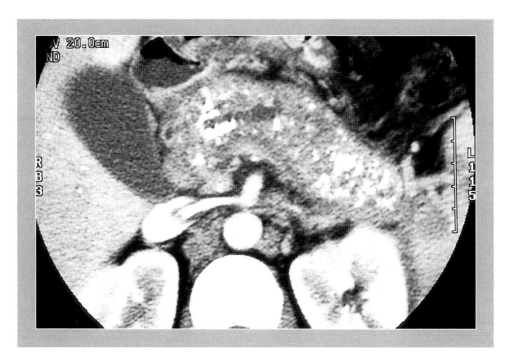

Figure 5.5 *Chronic pancreatitis* Abdominal CT scan of a heavy alcohol drinker who developed recurrent episodes of pancreatitis while on nebulized pentamidine (the only *Pneumocystis* prophylactic agent he could tolerate). The scan shows chronic calcific pancreatic disease

HEPATIC STEATOSIS

Risk factors for HAART-associated hepatic steatosis include weight > 70 kg, female sex and black African ethnicity. Its presentation can be extremely non-specific and symptoms will typically progress over several days. A blood lactate should be performed as an urgent investigation. Ultrasonography is a sensitive, accurate, non-invasive screening tool to detect steatosis as this is not always shown in liver function tests. Figure 5.6 shows the liver biopsy of an African patient with hepatic steatosis.

AVASCULAR NECROSIS

There are a growing number of reports of avascular necrosis among people with HIV. The most commonly affected bone is the femoral head, although it can also affect the shoulder or knee (Figure 5.7a and b). It may be asymptomatic or present with insidious pain. In up to 75% of cases it is bilateral. The cause of HIV-related avascular necrosis is not known. It is seen in both adults and children. In the latter case, the presentation is typically with hip pain or a limp. There is a strong association with systemic corticosteroid use (even when taken for just a few days). Some reports implicate hyperlipidemia as well as other drugs such as testosterone and HAART. Why avascular necrosis should be so common (up to 5% in one large series) is unclear, although it may be linked to the metabolic abnormalities discussed in the section concerning mitochondrial toxicity (p. 109). MRI scanning is an important diagnostic test as plain radiology is invariably normal.

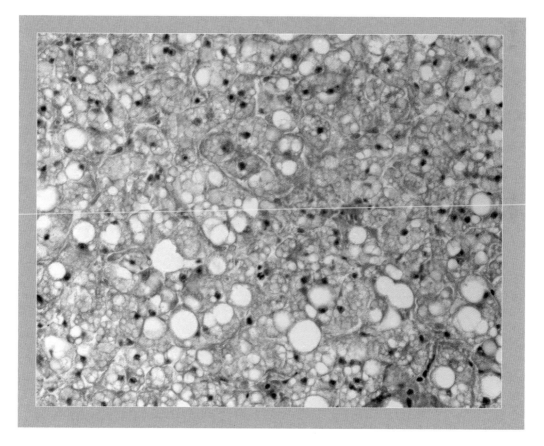

Figure 5.6 *Hepatic steatosis (H&E stain)* Liver biopsy from an African patient who had been taking antiretroviral therapy for several months and presented with a 2-week history of progressive nausea, malaise, abdominal pain and confusion associated with a deterioration in liver function tests. There is massive accumulation of fat within the hepatocytes, which are seen as clear spaces following sample processing. Despite discontinuation of HAART and aggressive supportive treatment, the patient became progressively more encephalopathic and died. The mechanism of this phenomenon is similar to that seen in Reye's syndrome in which children develop post-viral mitochondrial dysfunction, often associated with the use of aspirin. Encephalopathy results from hypoxic nerve cell damage and cerebral edema

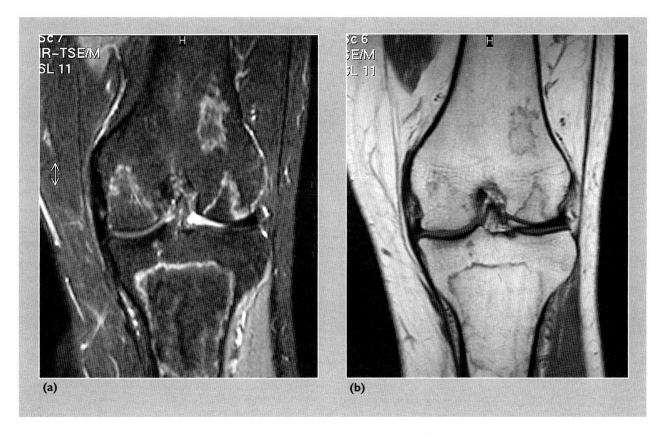

Figure 5.7 *Avascular necrosis* These knee MRI scans (**a**, T_1-weighted and **b**, T_2 STIR sequence) are from a young adult female who had been taking HAART for 3 months, and had presented with cerebral tuberculosis 2 months prior to this MR scan, for which she had received steroids as well as antimycobacterial therapy. She complained of slowly worsening pain in both knees. Plain radiological films were normal. The MRI scans show geographic, well-demarcated areas which have a fat signal intensity (**a**) and also surrounding edema (**b**). These are present in both the metaphyseal and subchondral regions of the knee. The features are characteristic of bone infarcts

High levels of osteopenia and osteoporosis have been reported in HIV-infected individuals. Some debate currently concerns the true prevalence of these conditions, although estimates would be along the lines of 30% and 15%, respectively. Risk factors for bone disease are lower pre-treatment body mass index (BMI), use of PIs and central obesity. Cohort studies in patients on HAART indicate that the rate of bone loss is related to the degree of co-existent lipoatrophy. If there is evidence that bone loss is occurring (e.g. malabsorption of vitamin D, hypogonadism, heavy alcohol or cigarette consumption or marked fat wasting on PIs), then DEXA bone scanning and vitamin D plus calcium levels should be performed.

MUSCULOSKELETAL DISEASE

Joint disease is common. It is often associated with Reiter's syndrome, in which it presents as a large joint asymmetric polyarticular arthritis of the lower limbs (up to 5% of sexually active patients). Patients are often HLA-B27 positive (75% of cases). Chlamydial infection has been implicated and it is reasonable to treat for this. Other causes of arthritis include psoriasis, HIV-associated arthritis (usually oligoarticular lower limb arthritis of uncertain cause, typically HLA-B27 negative), and painful articular syndrome. Septic arthritis and osteomyelitis are no more common than in the general population. Rheumatoid arthritis is rarely seen in HIV-infected individuals. The PI, indinavir, has been associated with an adhesive capsulitis known as 'frozen shoulder'.

Muscle disease can be pyogenic in origin (e.g. Staphylococcal pyomyositis), inflammatory (dermatomyositis) or drug-related. The muscle disease associated with zidovudine is part of the mitochondrial toxicity syndrome. Biopsy reveals the ragged red fibers characteristic of mitochondrial-damaged muscle.

RENAL DISEASE

HIV-associated nephropathy

As patients are living longer, there has been an increasing recognition of HIV-associated renal disease. It is now the third most common indication for dialysis among blacks between 20 and 64 years of age in the USA. It is more frequently seen in men and those of African ancestry. In the USA, it is estimated that up to 1 in 10 of such HIV-infected individuals have evidence of renal disease. The mechanism for this is unclear but probably relates to the direct effects of HIV proteins with consequent cytokine induction in renal structures. Concurrent hepatitis C infection is an additional risk factor.

Patients usually present with nephrotic syndrome (hypoalbuminemia and marked proteinuria) and progressive renal insufficiency. The most common lesion is so-called HIV-associated nephropathy (HIVAN). It is a glomerulopathy demonstrating focal segmental glomerulosclerosis (FSGS) with collapsing features (Figures 5.8 and 5.9).

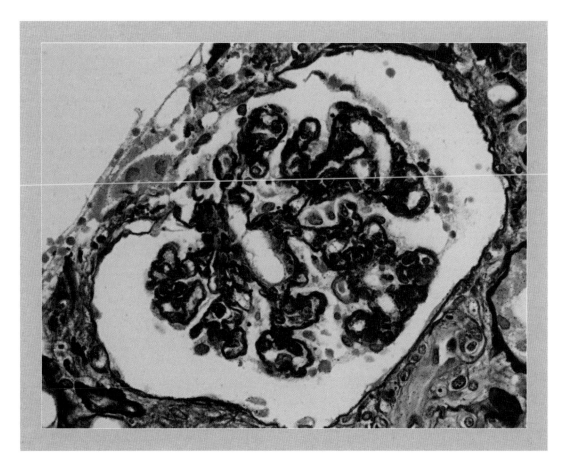

Figure 5.8 *Renal biopsy of HIV-associated nephropathy (PAMS stain)* This renal biopsy is that from a black African patient who complained of weakness and fatigue. Biochemically, she had moderately impaired renal function and was passing 4 g of protein per day. The image (periodic acid methenamine silver (PAMS) stain) shows the outlines of collapsing (wrinkled) capillary loops together with prominence of the visceral epithelial cells. These features are characteristic of early HIVAN

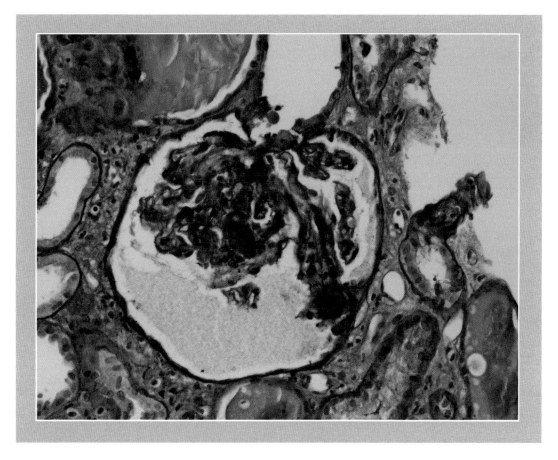

Figure 5.9 *HIV-associated nephropathy (PAS stain)* A more advanced case of renal disease is shown in a patient who required dialysis at presentation. There is marked sclerosis of the glomerular tuft. HIVAN, traditionally associated with a poor prognosis and rapid progression to end-stage renal disease within 3–6 months, at least in part responds to HAART and ACE inhibitors

As many as one-third of HIV-infected patients with renal disease who undergo renal biopsy will have other glomerular diseases, including membranoproliferative glomerulonephritis, minimal change disease, membranous glomerulopathy, amyloidosis, immune-complex glomerulonephritis and IgA nephropathy. The last is more common in white subjects. Biopsy is often, therefore, helpful to establish the correct diagnosis. Medication (including pentamidine, foscarnet, aminoglycosides, amphotericin B, ethambutol, indinavir, tenofovir and adefovir) as well as heroin can also produce renal disease, as may syphilis (Figure 5.10).

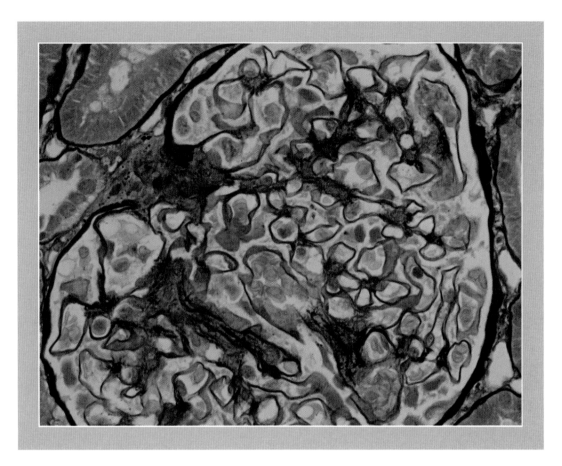

Figure 5.10 *HIV syphilitic membranous glomerulonephritis (PAMS stain)* This renal biopsy is from an HIV-infected white male who complained of a widespread rash associated with mild arthralgia. He had had recent unprotected sexual contacts, and was syphilis IgM antibody positive. He was found to have 6 g proteinuria, but otherwise normal renal function. The PAMS stain shows a near-normal glomerulus with only isolated pits seen where the capillary loop basement membrane is viewed obliquely. Electron microscopy revealed the subepithelial electron dense deposits that are found in membranous glomerulonephritis – the lesion typically associated with syphilis

6

Neurological disease

INTRODUCTION

Neurological disease is common. It can range from mild peripheral neuropathy with intermittent sensory symptoms to life-threatening intracerebral tumor or opportunistic infection. Ten per cent of HIV-positive patients present with a neurological AIDS-defining event. Overall, at least 50% of individuals with advanced HIV disease develop some form of neurological illness.

OPPORTUNISTIC CNS INFECTIONS

Opportunistic central nervous system (CNS) infection can present with either focal features or as diffuse neurological dysfunction. It is typically found in patients with CD4 counts $< 100 \times 10^6/l$. Over 90% of focal cerebral lesions are due to toxoplasmosis, primary CNS (PCNS) lymphoma, tuberculosis or progressive multifocal leukoencephalopathy. Clinically, these may be indistinguishable. Typical presentations include features suggesting a space-occupying mass lesion, such as hemiparesis or fits, or with non-specific symptoms of confusion, headache and fever. Other rarer causes of focal disease include bacterial abscess, viral infection (e.g. CMV, HSV), cryptococcoma, and cerebrovascular disease. It is important to remember that *Toxoplasma* is the most common and most easily treatable cause of focal lesions.

Diffuse cerebral dysfunction may manifest as drowsiness, confusion or behavioral changes. The most common infective cause is cryptococcal meningitis. This is seen in 5–10% of all patients with severe opportunistic infections. There is often little associated meningism. CSF and blood cryptococcal antigen are positive in > 90% of patients with cryptococcal meningitis while CSF India-ink stain for fungi is positive in only 70–80% with the disease. Blood cryptococcal antigen is therefore a useful screen in patients in whom clinical suspicion is low or lumbar puncture is contraindicated. However, all patients with CD4 counts $< 200 \times 10^6/l$ who present with fits, headache and fever, or confusion, should undergo cranial imaging. This can be either a CT or MRI scan, to exclude a space-occupying lesion that may be causing significant raised intracranial pressure. If safe to proceed, this should be followed by CSF examination. The investigation of such patients is summarized in Figure 6.1.

CSF examination can assist in the diagnosis of both neurological and febrile illness. The fluid should be examined cytologically (for cells and differential count, lymphoma, mycobacteria, fungi and viral inclusions), serologically (for neurosyphilis and *Cryptococcus*), biochemically (glucose and protein) and cultured for viruses, bacteria, mycobacteria and fungi. The recent introduction of nucleic acid amplification tests for viruses (HIV, the herpes family, JC virus – the cause of progressive multifocal leukoencephalopthy), bacteria (including mycobacteria) and protozoa (*Toxoplasma*) provides a further level of pathogen detection. These tests range between high sensitivity but poor specificity for active infection (e.g. Epstein–Barr virus) and the converse (e.g. *Toxoplasma*). A positive result must be interpreted in the clinical context in which it has been performed.

DRUG-INDUCED CNS DISEASE

A similar clinical picture of global CNS dysfunction can result from drug use (both prescribed and recreational) and systemic conditions (e.g. hypoxia or hepatic failure). Antiretroviral agents such as the nucleoside reverse transcriptase inhibitors (NRTIs), for example, stavudine, lamivudine and didanosine, have been implicated in the encephalopathy associated with hepatic steatosis and mitochondrial toxicity. The non-nucleoside RTI (NNRTI), efavirenz, will produce 'minor' CNS side-effects (insomnia, mood changes, depersonalization and depression) in up to 50% of individuals. A proportion of these (5–20%) will be severe enough to warrant drug cessation.

HIV NEUROPATHIC EFFECTS

Direct HIV infection of cells within the nervous system occurs early in the course of disease. Although often asymptomatic, this is demonstrated by the typical CSF findings of a slightly elevated protein, normal cellularity or mild mononuclear pleocytosis and normal glucose concentration. Occasionally, self-limiting meningoencephalitis and inflammatory neuropathies are seen during HIV seroconversion.

AIDS dementia complex

AIDS dementia complex (ADC), also known as HIV encephalopathy or HIV-associated dementia, occurs with advancing immunosuppression and is seen in up to 15% of symptomatic adults and 25% of children. Although its incidence has declined with the introduction of HAART by up to 50%, this is much less than the reductions noted in many of the other AIDS-defining illnesses. It may be that the incidence of ADC had already diminished with the widespread use of monotherapy or dual therapy containing zidovudine, prior to the introduction of HAART. The penetration of antiretroviral drugs may not be as effective in the CNS as it is at other sites such as the lung and gut. Opportunistic infections could therefore have fallen to a lesser extent within the brain compared to other organ systems.

The effect of antiretrovirals on the developing brain is an important area of research, since HIV-infected mothers now routinely receive medication during pregnancy. Whether this also leads to a reduction in HIV-related neurological disease (or other consequences) in the child is unclear.

ADC presents as a subcortical dementia with predominantly cognitive decline and symmetrical motor impairment. The history is typically several months in duration. Symptoms range from mild abnormalities on neuropsychometric testing associated with minor functional deficits, through depression or frank psychosis to severe cognitive dysfunction with paraparesis and incontinence. Children may present with expressive difficulties, attention deficits and hyperactivity. These do not necessarily progress to clear-cut dementia. Patients with ADC can function normally until an intercurrent infection unmasks their underlying disease. When the acute infection is treated, some of the clinical features may resolve. Therefore, patients presenting with cognitive impairment should always be thoroughly investigated for other causes of central nervous system disease. Furthermore, the radiological finding of cerebral atrophy does not necessarily correlate with the degree of clinical disability, and, in general, radiology is used to rule out other conditions that may give rise to similar symptoms, rather than confirming ADC.

Vacuolar myelopathy

Vacuolar myelopathy is probably due to direct HIV infection. It is seen in 25% of AIDS patients who undergo autopsy, although its clinical presentation as a spastic paraparesis without a definite sensory level is less common.

Peripheral neuropathy

Peripheral neuropathy is a common manifestation of HIV infection (found in 25% cases) and may occur in early or late disease. Typically, it presents in advanced HIV infection as a distal symmetrical sensory neuropathy. Occasionally, this will be functionally disabling (due more to pain than weakness). Distinctions must be made from drug-related neuropathies (e.g. due to the NRTIs such as zidovudine, didanosine, stavudine, zalcitabine, mycobacterial agents, such as isoniazid, or chemotherapy, such as vincristine) and CMV polyradiculopathy.

Mononeuritis multiplex and autonomic neuropathy

A severe form of mononeuritis multiplex and autonomic neuropathy may be found in patients with advanced disease. The latter can produce disabling postural hypotension and contribute to chronic diarrhea. Rarely, subacute inflammatory demyelinating neuropathy is seen at an earlier stage of HIV infection. This presents with weakness and depressed tendon jerks. Unlike the later sensory neuropathy or vacuolar myelopathy, the outcome here is generally good. It should be noted that dramatic improvements have been seen with HAART and that a trial of antiretroviral therapy is often warranted in patients with documented neuropathy. Drugs with least chance of producing similar side-effects to the clinical complaint should be selected, although even if this is not possible, the benefits may still outweigh the disadvantages.

Myopathy

Muscle pain and weakness can occur at all stages of HIV infection. Proximal myopathy is commonly due to HIV infection or medication (e.g. NRTIs such as zidovudine). However, weakness may also result from general debility and loss of muscle bulk rather than intrinsic muscle disease. In true myopathy, serum creatine kinase will usually be elevated and electromyography will be abnormal.

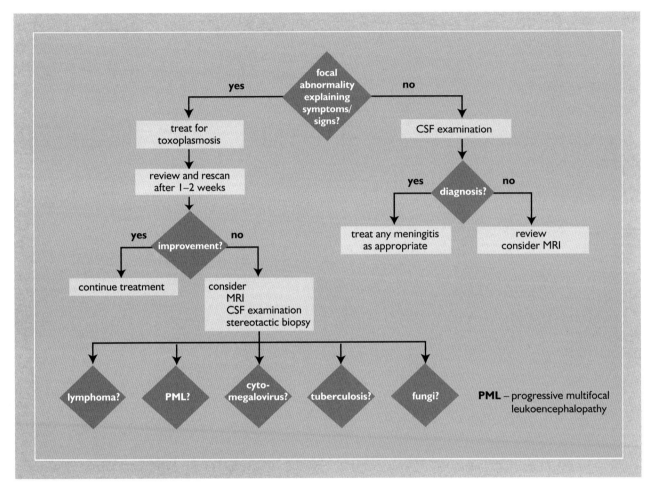

Figure 6.1 Diagnostic algorithm based on the results of a cranial CT scan. Note that the chance of toxoplasmosis is less if the patient has a history of regular use of co-trimoxazole or is toxoplasma lgG-negative. Hence, early review is recommended in such individuals

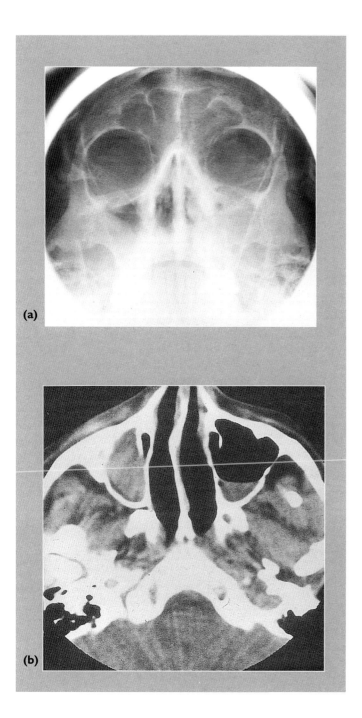

(a)

(b)

Figure 6.2 *Sinus disease* This may present as headache and fever with or without localizing features of facial pain, post-nasal drip or nasal congestion. It should, therefore, be considered as a differential diagnosis of meningitis. Sinusitis is often chronic (predominantly in patients with low CD4 counts). It can be complicated by acute infective exacerbations and orbital or intracranial extension. Bacterial pathogens responsible include *Streptococcus pneumoniae*, *Hemophilus influenzae* and *Pseudomonas aeruginosa*. Non-resolution or worsening symptoms of an acute episode should be investigated by sinus aspiration or antral washout. Unusual organisms include fungi, protozoa and complex bacteria. Plain sinus radiography can provide an indication of the extent of disease. Normal radiographs make sinusitis unlikely. However, it has poor specificity such that individuals with no sinus disease can have apparently abnormal radiology. **(a)** A completely opaque left maxillary sinus, and severe mucosal thickening on the right is shown. CT scanning may provide more detail and is important if a patient is not improving on standard treatment. In **(b)** the right antrum is opaque and there is fluid in the left maxillary sinus. The patient also had sphenoidal and fronto-ethmoidal involvement. CT scans can indicate the presence of subtle bony abnormalities, which can be helpful if there is a concern about invasive disease. MRI scanning is also useful, although rarely adds much (beyond reducing the amount of radiation a patient receives) in this context

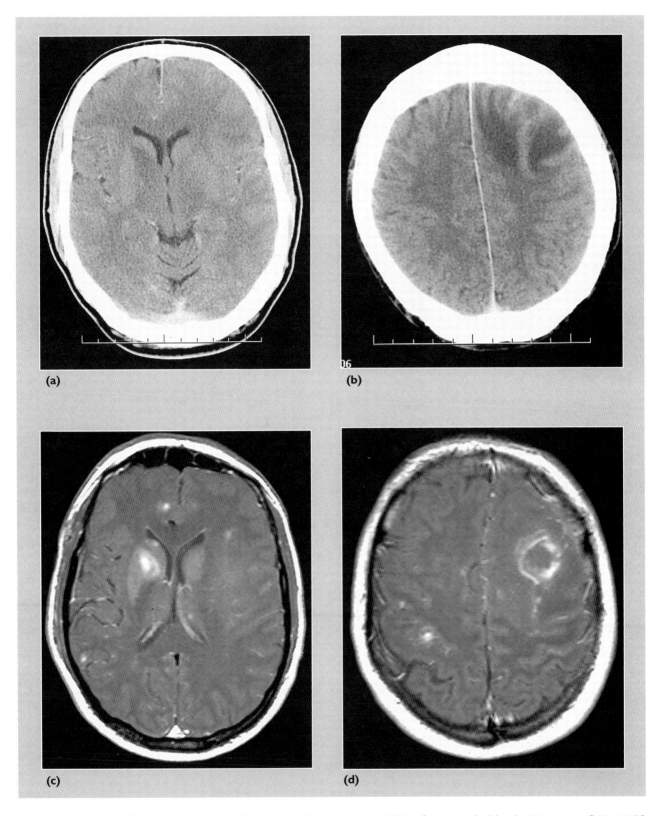

Figure 6.3 *Toxoplasmosis* **(a and b)** CT brain scans of a patient with HIV infection and a blood CD4 count of 40 x 10⁶/l who presented with expressive dysphasia, headache and fever. The scans show subtle low-density changes in the right anterior internal capsule and loss of the medial lentiform nucleus; together with a mixed signal in the left frontal lobe **(b)**. The MR scans **(c and d)** confirm these findings and also reveal further frontal and temporoparietal lesions

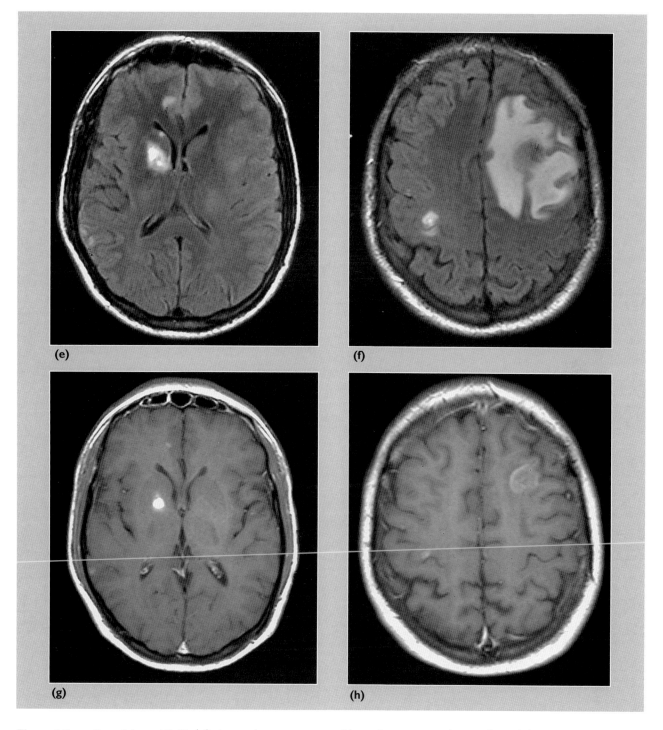

Figure 6.3 continued (e and f) Gadolinium enhancement is visible in these scans, indicating loss of the normal blood–brain barrier. The patient was started empirically on anti-*Toxoplasma* therapy together with oral corticosteroids. His dysphasia improved over the next 3 days, although transiently worsened at days 4 and 5. A blood nucleic acid amplification test (PCR) for *Toxoplasma* was positive. His recovery continued and a repeat MR scan at week 4 of treatment revealed a reduction in the size of the ring-enhancing lesions (**g and h**; T_1-weighted image post-gadolinium). The acute mortality of cerebral toxoplasmosis is about 10%. A further 25% of patients are left with some residual neurological deficit. The differential diagnosis of cerebral mass lesions included toxoplasmosis, lymphoma – typically PCNS, tuberculosis and other infections.

The CT and MR scans demonstrate the technical superiority of MRI particularly in the detection of posterior fossa lesions. Apart from lack of availability of MR scanning in some centers, the main limitation to its use is the presence of metal implants within the patient such as an aneurysm clip or a pacemaker which could be displaced by the scanner's powerful magnetic field

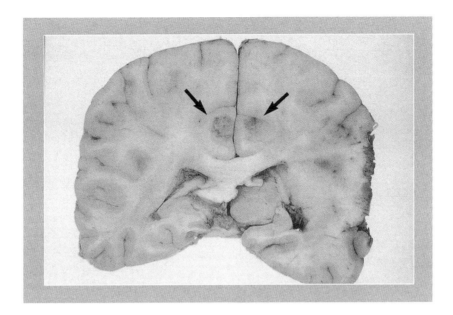

Figure 6.4 *Cerebral toxoplasmosis* Up to 10% of patients with toxoplasmosis will present with a diffuse encephalitis, and no focal symptoms. CSF examination is typically unhelpful. A therapeutic response to empirical treatment will be clinically evident in 90% of cases after 1 week. Radiological improvement is apparent in almost all patients with toxoplasmosis at the end of 2 weeks. If a tissue diagnosis is required, CT- or MRI-guided stereotactic biopsy is the investigation of choice. This enables a definitive diagnosis to be made in up to 90% of cases, and can reveal dual pathology within one lesion (5%). There is a low perioperative morbidity. The coronal slice of the brain shows lesions in the medial surface of both hemispheres caused by *Toxoplasma*. Scarring is evident on the surface of one hemisphere at the site of an open brain biopsy, a procedure no longer recommended

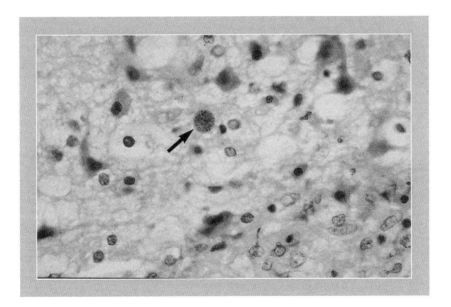

Figure 6.5 *Cerebral toxoplasmosis (H&E stain)* Inflammatory changes in the brain are seen due to *Toxoplasma*. A *Toxoplasma* cyst is also present. In 95% of cases, acute cerebral toxoplasmosis reflects a reactivation of previous quiescent infection. This occurs when CD4 counts are usually $< 100 \times 10^6/l$. Positive serology is a common finding in the general population and therefore the presence of immunoglobulin G (IgG) cannot distinguish between active disease and other causes of space-occupying lesions. The level of circulating IgG *Toxoplasma* antibody in a patient with no evidence of acute disease can predict those at risk of reactivation, although the onset of clinical disease may be several years after the increase in antibody titer (relative risk increased by a factor of 3.6 if antibody > 150 IU/ml). Patients with no serological evidence of exposure to *Toxoplasma* should be advised to avoid primary infection from animals (typically ingestion of oocysts from cat feces present in cat litter or soil) or uncooked meat (pork or lamb)

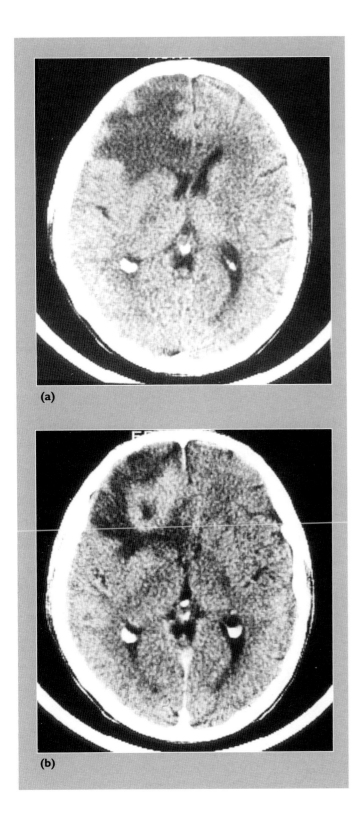

(a)

(b)

Figure 6.6   *Single mass lesion*   The CT scans, **(a)** plain and **(b)** with contrast, show a large right frontal contrast-enhancing lesion with associated edema and mass effect. This radiological appearance is typically due to cerebral toxoplasmosis or PCNS lymphoma. This patient, with a CD4 count of $< 50 \times 10^6$/l, was started empirically on anti-*Toxoplasma* treatment but after 2 weeks there was no clinical or radiological improvement. Stereotactic biopsy was performed and demonstrated PCNS lymphoma. The patient received cranial irradiation but died within 6 weeks.

HIV-related PCNS lymphoma will manifest radiologically as either single or multiple (50–70% cases) hypodense contrast-enhancing lesions. These are often present in a periventricular or meningeal distribution. Lesions may enhance homogenously, although are often thick-walled cavities. These can be difficult to distinguish from other causes of intracerebral abscess, such as toxoplasmosis, which can present as a solitary mass up to 40% of the time. However, while the latter responds well to therapy, the prognosis for PCNS lymphoma is poor. Toxoplasmosis treatment trials remain a justifiable approach, although this diagnosis is much less likely if the patient has a history of regular co-trimoxazole use for *Pneumocystis* prophylaxis (which provides good protection against toxoplasmosis reactivation), or is *Toxoplasma* IgG antibody-negative in serum. Brain biopsy would then be indicated if there was a poor response to therapy or persistently negative *Toxoplasma* serology after 1–2 weeks in a patient with previous good quality of life

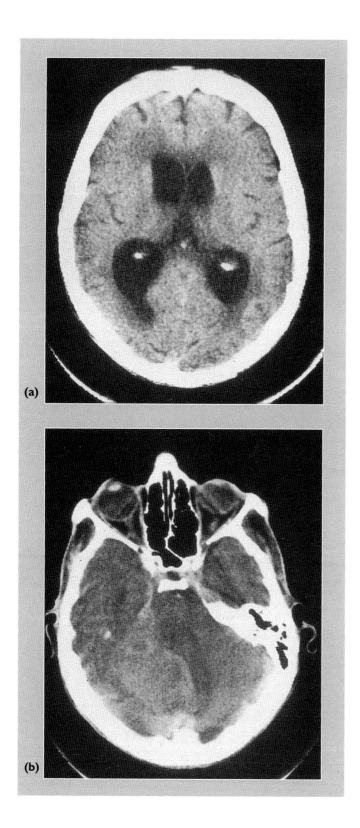

(a)

(b)

Figure 6.7 *Primary CNS lymphoma producing hydrocephalus* The CT scan **(a)** reveals marked dilatation of the lateral ventricles. This is the appearance of supratentorial hydrocephalus and resulted from obstruction of the 4th ventricle by a substantial mass in the right cerebellar hemisphere which showed irregular patchy enhancement **(b)**. The patient presented with headache, gross ataxia and incontinence. He declined investigation or treatment

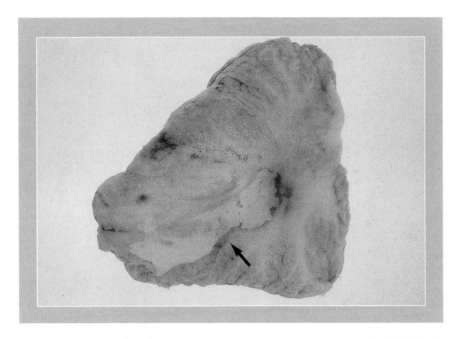

Figure 6.7 continued *Primary CNS lymphoma* **(c)** Postmortem examination revealed PCNS B-cell non-Hodgkin's lymphoma (arrow) involving the cerebellum. Posterior fossa masses can present with acute hydrocephalus, and symptomatic relief may be obtained by ventricular shunting.

In cases of suspected PCNS lymphoma, CSF sampling can be helpful. Although cytology for lymphomatous cells is usually negative (at least 70% of cases), Epstein–Barr virus PCR will be positive in over 80%. Thus, a negative result should prompt consideration of other diagnoses. The use of non-invasive imaging such as thallium-210 single-photon emission CT (SPECT) may help to differentiate lymphoma from infectious intracerebral disease, since tumor cells take up isotope to a greater extent

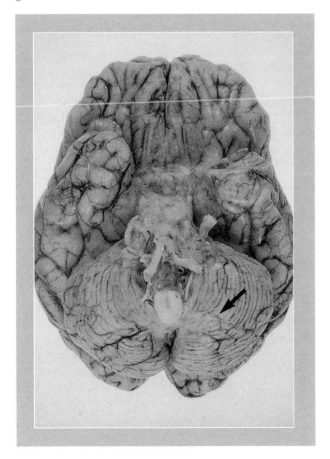

Figure 6.8 *Leptomeningeal opacities due to tuberculous meningitis* The resurgence of tuberculosis associated with HIV has led to a recent increase in the incidence of tuberculous meningitis (arrow). The clinical presentation and CSF findings of HIV-related tuberculous meningitis are similar to those seen in an immunocompetent population. In about 50% of cases, this is associated with extrameningeal disease

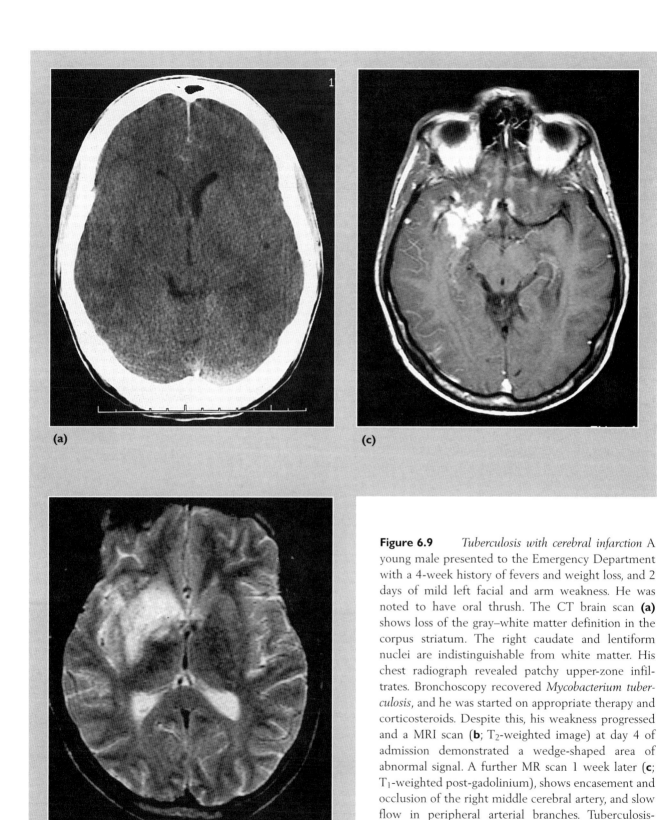

(a)

(c)

(b)

Figure 6.9 *Tuberculosis with cerebral infarction* A young male presented to the Emergency Department with a 4-week history of fevers and weight loss, and 2 days of mild left facial and arm weakness. He was noted to have oral thrush. The CT brain scan (**a**) shows loss of the gray–white matter definition in the corpus striatum. The right caudate and lentiform nuclei are indistinguishable from white matter. His chest radiograph revealed patchy upper-zone infiltrates. Bronchoscopy recovered *Mycobacterium tuberculosis*, and he was started on appropriate therapy and corticosteroids. Despite this, his weakness progressed and a MRI scan (**b**; T_2-weighted image) at day 4 of admission demonstrated a wedge-shaped area of abnormal signal. A further MR scan 1 week later (**c**; T_1-weighted post-gadolinium), shows encasement and occlusion of the right middle cerebral artery, and slow flow in peripheral arterial branches. Tuberculosis-associated cerebral infarction is a consequence of the vasculitis that accompanies the disease. It is more common in HIV-related mycobacterial infection

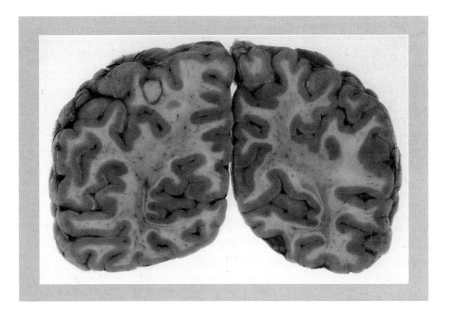

Figure 6.10   *Tuberculous abscess* The postmortem specimen shows a tuberculous abscess in the left cerebral hemisphere. There were also lesions within the cerebellum. It is rare to see posterior fossa disease in toxoplasmosis, and this can be a useful way of distinguishing the two conditions if radiology demonstrates disease at that anatomical site. Lesions that have a low signal ring on MRI T_2-weighted images (without contrast) are more typically due to tuberculosis. CSF sampling may be helpful as tuberculosis spreads from the brain substance into the CSF, giving rise to features of tuberculosis meningitis

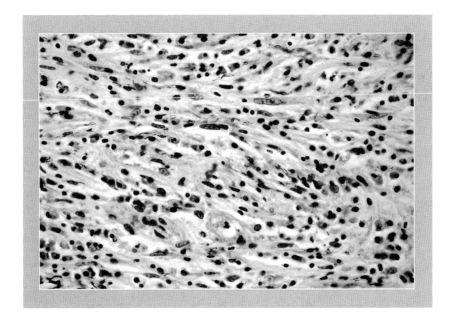

Figure 6.11   *Tuberculoma* This sample is from an African teenager who had previously been treated for tuberculosis, but had been lost to follow-up after 4 months of therapy. She presented 12 months later with a short history of headache and collapse. A brain scan indicated a large cerebral mass lesion causing raised intracranial pressure. The brain biopsy with ZN staining shows numerous red-staining acid fast bacilli. The patient was found to be HIV-positive and, despite aggressive therapy, died. HIV testing should be offered to all patients with tuberculosis. Antiretroviral therapy reduces the 1-year risk of death from 20% to less than 5%

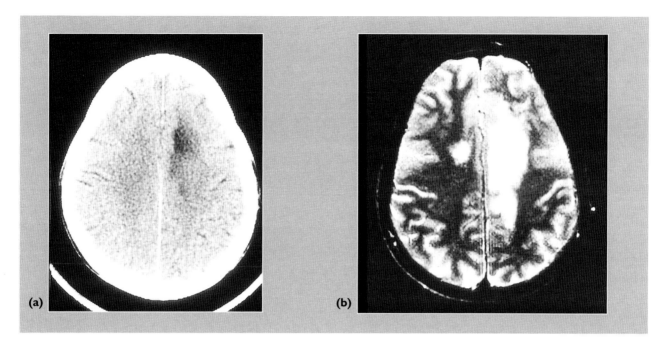

Figure 6.12   *Progressive multifocal leukoencephalopathy (PML)* The patient presented with a sudden onset of nominal dysphasia. A CT scan **(a)** demonstrated a lesion at the watershed between anterior and middle cerebral artery territories, suggesting an underlying vascular cause. However, cerebral angiography was normal. The patient became confused and aphasic and T₂-weighted MRI **(b)** revealed extensive white matter disease in both hemispheres – the typical features of PML. The disease presents with focal deficits in the absence of fever and progresses within weeks to severe cerebral dysfunction and death. CT scanning shows hypodense lesions which only rarely enhance with contrast, and do not exert mass effect. This case illustrates the advantages of MRI in situations where CT brain scanning does not explain the clinical picture

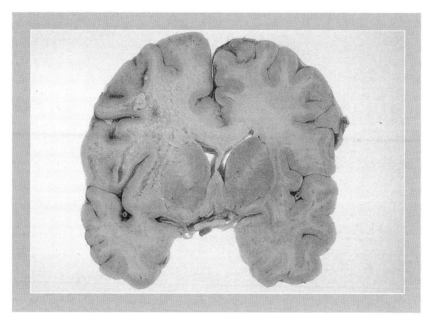

Figure 6.13   *Progressive multifocal leukoencephalopathy (PML)* The coronal slice of the cerebral hemisphere shows striking degeneration of the left parietal lobe white matter. The cortical gray matter is spared. This subacute demyelinating disease is seen in up to 1% of AIDS patients and a further 3% at postmortem. Other demyelinating processes that can give a similar picture to PML include acute disseminated encephalomyelitis (ADEM) and multiple sclerosis. Both of these are characterized by multifocal white matter involvement, and present with diffuse neurological signs together with multifocal lesions in the brain and spinal cord. ADEM is probably a T-cell mediated autoimmune response to myelin basic protein, triggered by an infection (including HIV) or vaccination, and may respond to HAART

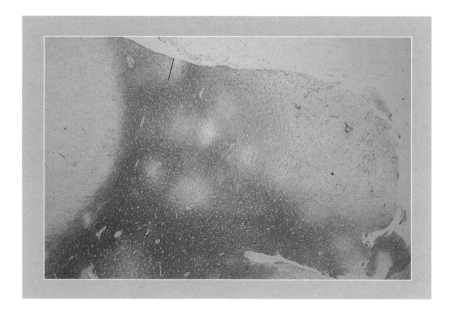

Figure 6.14   *Progressive multifocal leukoencephalopathy (PML)* Infection with JC virus (a papova virus) has resulted in patchy pale areas of demyelination within the cerebral hemisphere (LFB stain). The diagnosis of PML is often made by a combination of clinical and radiographic features. However, the evolving spectrum of opportunistic pathogens means that more brain biopsies are now performed. Here, JC virus may be demonstrable using *in situ* hybridization or nucleic acid amplification (PCR) techniques. CSF is PCR-positive in 50–90% of cases

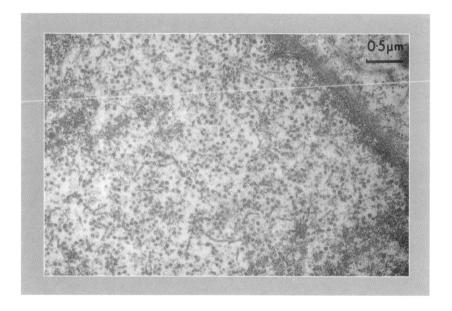

Figure 6.15   *Progressive multifocal leukoencephalopathy (PML)* An electron micrograph from a postmortem brain specimen demonstrating intranuclear virus particles resembling JC virus in a patient with PML. The outlook for untreated PML is poor, with typical survival being 4–6 months. Factors associated with an improved outlook include CD4 count > 100 x 10⁶/l at diagnosis, use of (and response to) HAART, lack of brainstem involvement and low baseline JC CSF viral load. HAART appears to halt PML in 70% of subjects and improves neurological findings in one-half of these cases

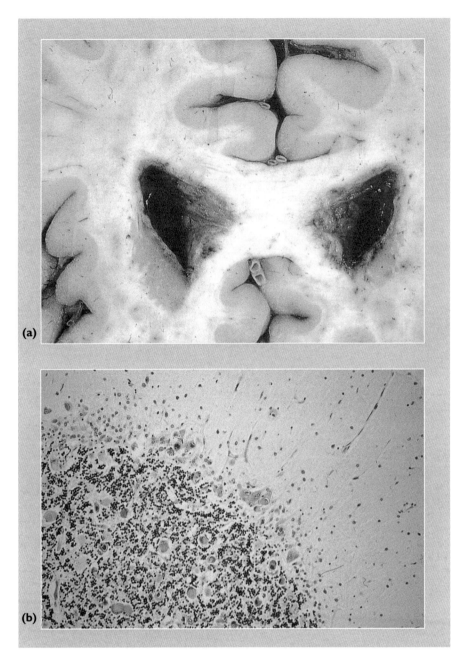

Figure 6.16 *CMV encephalitis* CMV infection in the brain is a common finding at postmortem (25% of AIDS patients) and, in a proportion of these people, it causes an encephalitis with progressive drowsiness, brainstem signs and seizures. Often the CT scan will be normal, the MRI non-specific (periventricular enhancement or, occasionally, ring-enhancing focal lesions) and EEG usually unhelpful. Blood and CSF cultures add little, although CSF PCR has a high sensitivity and specificity (80–90%). Although concomitant opportunistic CNS infection is common, a trial of anti-CMV therapy is appropriate in patients with an undiagnosed encephalitis, especially if they have a history of previous CMV disease or are PCR-positive in blood or CSF. **(a)** The ependymitis in the postmortem is typical – shown here in the anterior horns of the lateral ventricles. **(b)** The microscopic appearance of numerous CMV inclusions seen in both the Purkinje and granular cell layers of the cerebellum is demonstrated (H&E stain). Herpes simplex may also cause an encephalitis which may have a subacute and less focal presentation than in the non-immunosuppressed. Brain scanning and EEG may therefore lack the characteristic feature of predominant temporal lobe involvement found in the immunocompetent.

Varicella zoster virus (VZV) CNS infection in HIV is relatively rare, although typically produces a small vessel encephalitis following an episode of shingles. The latter may have been several months earlier, and should be specifically enquired about in the history. A CSF examination usually reveals mononuclear cells (< 1000, predominantly lymphocytes) and a mildly raised protein. PCR for VZV is useful

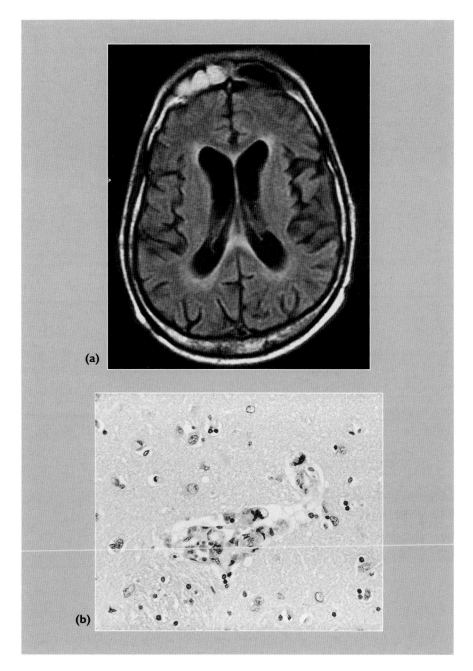

Figure 6.17   *AIDS dementia complex* The MR scan (**a**; T$_2$-weighted image with flair – CSF suppression) shows the typical appearance of cerebral atrophy – widened cerebral sulci and enlarged lateral ventricles with poorly defined hyperintensity in the periventricular white matter. These changes are also present on CT scanning, although they are non-specific and may be seen in many patients with no apparent cognitive, motor or behavioral deficits. MRI may also show patchy T$_2$-weighted abnormalities in the white matter, although it cannot distinguish between asymptomatic individuals and those with early AIDS dementia complex (ADC). In a patient with features of a subcortical dementia, radiology is used to rule out space-occupying mass lesions. The differential diagnosis of ADC includes CMV encephalitis, cryptococcal meningitis and neurosyphilis – all of which have non-specific CT/MR appearances. CSF examination is important and should include testing for these conditions. CSF findings in ADC are non-specific; often a few mononuclear cells are present together with a slight increase in protein. HIV load in CSF can be increased, as are β-2 microglobulin and quinolinic acid. The histopathological findings of white matter pallor and multinucleated giant cells (**b**), seen in the perivascular space in the basal ganglia, are found in most patients dying with ADC. Neuronal depletion is probably not due to direct HIV infection, but rather the result of brain macrophage infection. This leads to metabolic and cytokine dysregulation with subsequent neuron cell death by apoptosis. It is likely that this set of events is initiated outside the brain and results from cerebral invasion by macrophages. Consistent with this, risk factors for ADC include low blood CD4 count (< 200 x 10^6/l), wasting and anemia

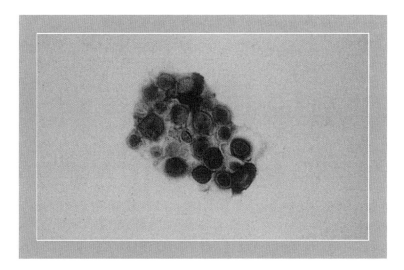

Figure 6.18 *Cryptococcal disease* The clinical picture of cryptococcal meningitis ranges from mild headache and fever to severe generalized cerebral dysfunction. It is responsible for almost 50% of cases of meningitis in the Southern hemisphere. Extracerebral disease involving typically the lung or skin is seen in 30% of cases. The CSF is often bland, although cryptococcal antigen is positive in blood or CSF in over 90% of infections. India-ink staining for organisms is positive in 75%. *Cryptococcus* organisms engulfed by a single macrophage within cerebrospinal fluid can be seen. Factors predicting a poor outcome include confusion, raised CSF opening pressure (> 25 cm) and CSF cryptoccal antigen titer > 1 : 1024. Changes in the latter value are not helpful when monitoring treatment response.

Bacteria are responsible for up to a quarter of all cases of meningitis in the developing world. Common organisms are *Streptococcus pneumoniae, Hemophilus influenzae* and *Neisseria meningitidis*. They present in a similar manner to that seen in HIV-negative individuals. Blood cultures are a useful investigation, and response to antibiotics is good. Although migrainous and tension headaches are seen within the HIV-positive population, one should have a low threshold for investigating headache in the immunocompromised

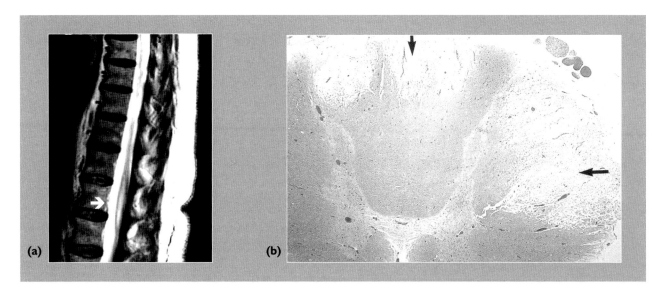

Figure 6.19 *Spinal cord disease* A patient presented with paraparesis and a thoracic sensory level. CT myelogram and examination of the CSF were unhelpful. Sagittal MRI **(a)** revealed a high signal intrinsic lesion expanding the mid-thoracic portion of the spinal cord (arrow). MRI scanning can precisely localize cord disease, but often provides little information on the exact etiology. Biopsy may then be indicated. Causes of a transverse myelitis include viruses (herpes zoster), bacterial, mycobacterial or *Toxoplasma* abscesses or intramedullary lymphoma.

Subacute or chronic progressive spinal cord disease is often due to HIV vacuolar myelopathy. **(b)** Vacuolation within the posterior and posterolateral columns of the thoracic spinal cord. The condition is usually associated with AIDS dementia complex and hence patients often have more diffuse clinical signs. Imaging of these cords as well as CSF examination is usually normal. Rarely HTLV-1 may produce a similar clinical picture and should be suspected when serology is positive

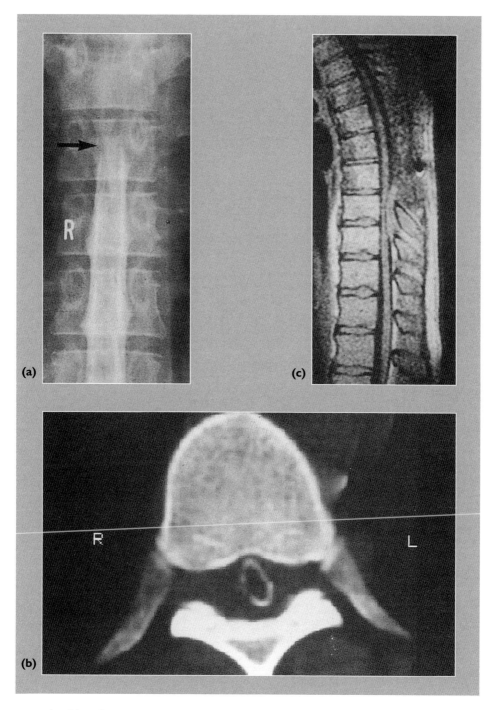

Figure 6.20 *Extradural lymphoma* A patient presented with a short history of back pain progressing to flaccid paraparesis, urinary retention and a sensory level. Myelography **(a)** revealed an obstruction to the flow of contrast in the mid-thoracic spine. There was no bony abnormality present. CT myelography at this level **(b)** showed that an extradural mass within the spinal canal was compressing the theca and cord. Emergency laminectomy and excision of a non-Hodgkin's lymphoma was performed. After a course of chemo- and radiotherapy, the patient's signs almost completely resolved. Ten months later he returned with recurrent symptoms. MRI (proton density) **(c)** revealed tumor recurrence compressing the dorsal aspect of the cord deep to the laminectomy

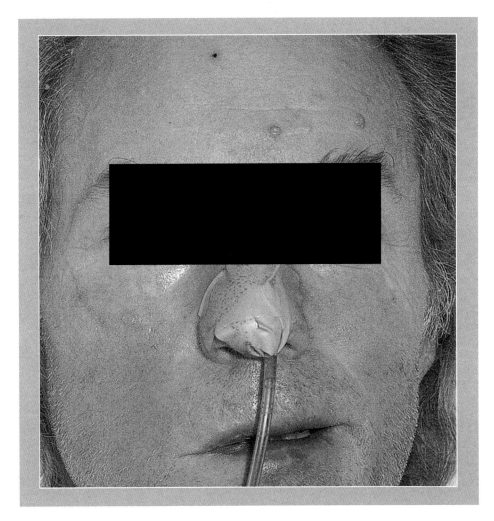

Figure 6.21 *Peripheral neuropathies* The patient presented with abdominal pain, vomiting, fever and a 7th nerve lesion. The illustration shows right facial weakness with loss of right forehead ridges and mild right parotid swelling. A nasogastric tube has been passed. The patient had lymphomatous involvement of the right parotid gland. In general, mononeuropathies (including cranial nerve palsy) arise from tumor infiltration, vasculitis or basal meningitis.

Peripheral neuropathies can be clinically classified as distal symmetric polyneuropathy (DSP), inflammatory demyelinating polyneuropathy (IDP), progressive polyradiculopathy (PP) and mononeuritis complex. DSP (typically numbness or burning in a glove and stocking distribution) occurs in up to 35% of patients. It is associated with high HIV loads, low CD4 counts, advanced disease and increasing age. DSP is clinically indistinguishable from the toxic neuropathy induced by drug therapies. Investigations should exclude other causes of DSP such as syphilis, hematinic deficiency states and thyroid disease. Mononeuritis and IDP are less common, although they can occur early in HIV infection. The latter presents with ascending weakness and little sensory involvement. CSF findings are a high protein and moderate lymphocyte infiltration. As in both mononeuritis and PP, which presents with pain in a cauda equina distribution together with loss of bowel and bladder function, it is important in IDP to exclude CMV infection. Other causes of PP are varicella zoster and lymphoma

7

Ocular disease

INTRODUCTION

Ophthalmic complications have been reported in up to 60% of HIV-infected individuals. These range from a mild transient viral conjunctivitis to sight-threatening retinitis. Full eye examination is important as any orbital tissue may be affected. External examination may reveal a palpable mass or proptosis caused by tumor. The eyelids can be infected by molluscum contagiosum. Slit-lamp examination of the conjunctiva distinguishes between inflammation due to a mild viral conjunctivitis and Kaposi's sarcoma. Inflammation in the anterior chamber and keratitic precipitates on the cornea indicate uveitis. This may be non-specific or due to medication. Thorough history-taking and retinal examination are paramount as severe disease may present initially as only a mild uveitis.

The increasing use of highly active antitretroviral therapy has had a major impact on ophthalmological practice with a fall in the incidence of severe opportunistic disease. There is, however, an associated drug toxicity. Stevens–Johnson syndrome, as well as toxic epidermal necrolysis, cause severe dry eyes which can lead to corneal ulceration, infection and loss of vision. A corneal vortex keratopathy has been described associated with lipophilic drugs such as aciclovir.

The most common severe ocular opportunistic infection in both the developing and developed world is cytomegalovirus (CMV) retinitis. This progressive, destructive condition is reported in up to 25% of individuals with advanced HIV disease. Untreated it will result in blindness. Although it appears to be less common in the developed world this may reflect 'competition' from other infections such as tuberculosis which occur at an earlier stage of HIV infection. WHO estimates that 10–20% of HIV-infected individuals will ultimately develop sight-threatening CMV disease, as prophylaxis for other conditions is implemented. Currently available drugs active against CMV delay progression but are not curative. CMV retinitis is best treated by restoration of the patient's specific immune competence. This is now a realistic objective, and HAART has led to an 80% reduction in the incidence of CMV disease.

The early stage of peripheral CMV retinitis is asymptomatic, although some patients may complain of floaters or a 'blank patch' as a result of a visual field defect. Late-stage CMV retinitis or a centrally placed lesion will cause a reduction in visual acuity. Untreated focal CMV retinitis doubles in size every month. Spread to the other eye is common, but can be averted by systemic treatment. CMV retinitis is often no longer a preterminal event – hence its treatment has important implications for long-term health status and disability.

Patients for whom HAART has not been successful or is unavailable, and who have CD4 counts $< 100 \times 10^6/l$ are susceptible to CMV retinitis. Asymptomatic individuals can be monitored with quantitative blood CMV DNA viral load. Persistently elevated titers imply an increased risk of end-organ disease. The relative hazard of developing retinitis in CMV DNA-positive patients compared to DNA-negative patients who are CMV-antibody positive is four times if CD4 $< 100 \times 10^6/l$ and 20 times if CD4 $< 50 \times 10^6/l$. Increased CMV viral load also predicts clinical disease. Each 0.25 log rise in CMV titer increases the risk by 40.

Patients with pre-existing CMV disease who commence HAART may be susceptible to immune recovery uveitis. This condition develops as the host's native cell function and antigen recognition are restored. It may manifest as vitritis, cystoid macular edema or an epiretinal membrane, all of which can impair vision. This has been reported in up to 15% of individuals with CMV retinitis who are starting antiretrovirals.

Severely immunocompromised patients are also susceptible to other conditions. An ischemic retinopathy is seen in between a third and a half of patients with symptomatic disease. This may be due to direct HIV infection. The microangiopathy produces retinal cotton wool spots which must be distinguished from early CMV retinitis.

Other opportunistic infections were rare even in the days before HAART was widely available, with an incidence of < 5%. They are now infrequently seen in the developed world. Eye involvement is usually a manifestation of systemic opportunistic infection and dissemination. *Toxoplasma gondii* and *Pneumocystis* can invade the choroid. Varicella zoster virus may cause an acute retinal necrosis. The incidence of ocular syphilis and tuberculosis reflects the prevalence in the general population from which patients are drawn.

Neuro-ophthalmic examination is able to identify cranial nerve palsies, which are the result of intracranial infections and neoplasms. Visual field defects without ocular pathology are indicative of a space-occupying lesion typically due to a *Toxoplasma* abscess or a lymphoma.

Patients with cryptococcal meningitis can develop papilledema or optic nerve papillitis. Deteriorating color vision without optic atrophy can occur. In such cases, the swelling is assumed to be due to primary HIV optic neuropathy, but it is important to consider drug toxicity, for example, as a result of the antituberculosis drug ethambutol.

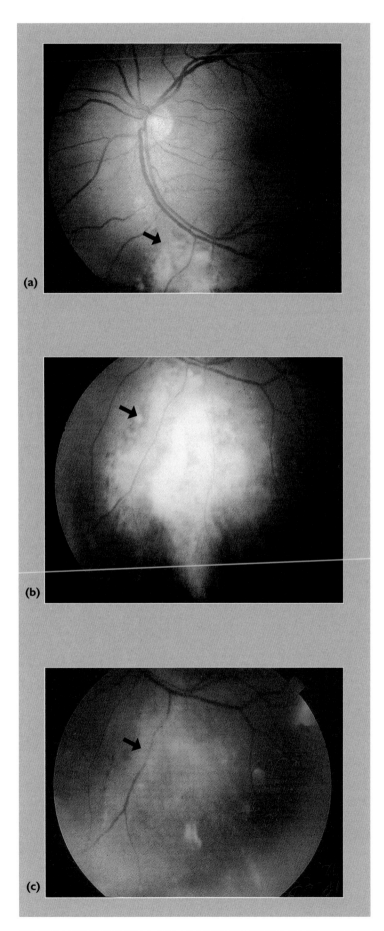

Figure 7.1 *Active CMV retinitis* **(a)** This photograph is from a patient who complained of a 'blank patch' in his right upper visual field, but with no loss of visual acuity. There is a diamond-shaped zone of white retinal necrosis (arrow) inferior to the temporal blood vessels. Four characteristic signs of CMV retinitis are shown in this example: white granular retinal opacification with ill-defined borders; associated hemorrhages mainly at the borders of the lesion; the lesion follows the contours of the blood vessels; and a low-grade vitritis (allowing easy retinal visualization) associated with extensive retinal necrosis. **(b)** The same patient looking down. This is a close-up view of the zone of white retinal necrosis (arrow). Following treatment, fundoscopy taken 6 weeks later **(c)** shows that the acute infection has resolved, leaving an area of pale, thin, retinal atrophy (arrow)

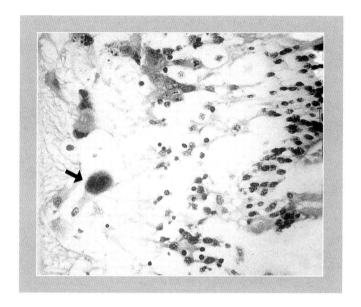

Figure 7.2   *Active CMV retinitis* Histology of CMV retinitis shows a CMV 'owl's-eye' inclusion (arrow) in the ganglion cell layer of the retina

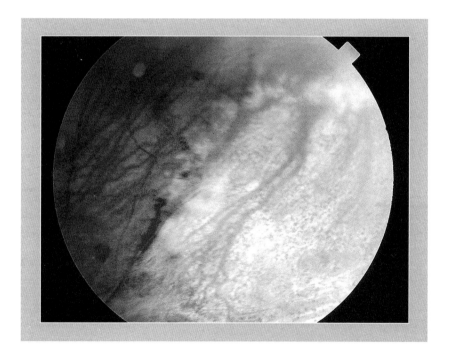

Figure 7.3   *Brushfire progression of CMV retinitis* Fundoscopy of untreated CMV retinitis reveals the characteristic brushfire progression of the condition. There is a leading edge of active disease spreading diagonally onto the unaffected retina, leaving atrophic tissue in its wake (lower right side of the field). Most CMV retinitis initially affects only one eye but, in 80% of patients, both eyes are eventually involved

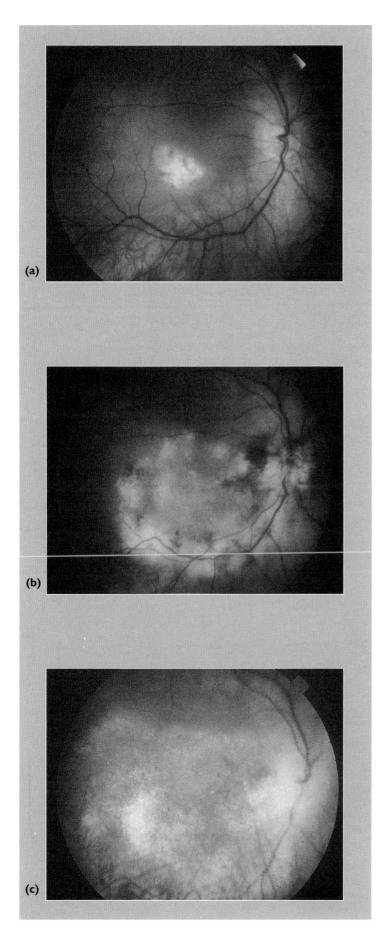

Figure 7.4 *Central CMV lesion with progression* **(a)** Fundoscopy of a patient who complained of distorted vision in his right eye. His visual acuity was normal. There is an area of white granular retinal necrosis with hemorrhage at the edge inferior to the fovea. **(b)** The same patient 4 months later. The previous lesion had responded to anti-CMV therapy, but the patient then presented with a rapid deterioration of his vision. The visual acuity of his right eye fell to 6/60. There is a lesion involving the inferior half of the macula which reaches the inferior temporal arcade and the optic disc. The central area is the original focus of treated CMV retinitis which is now atrophic. **(c)** The same patient, taken 3 months later. The CMV disease has healed, resulting in retinal and optic atrophy. The patient was blind in his right eye. Pre-HAART studies suggested that the median time to severe visual impairment (worse than 20/200) was 13 months from initial disease. However, many patients would have already died of other opportunistic events by then

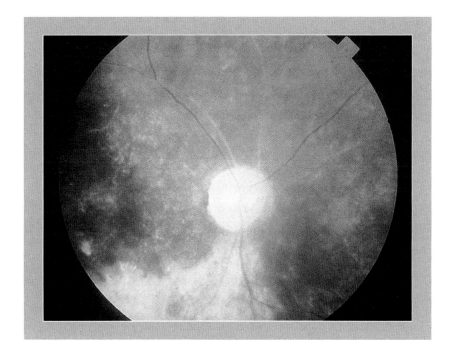

Figure 7.5   *Optic atrophy* Fundoscopy of optic atrophy shows a dense white optic disc; the emerging arteries are white and sclerosed. Along the inferior temporal vessels is a large, white, full-thickness, retinal necrotic scar. This is 'burnt-out' CMV retinitis which originally involved the optic disc, causing a papillitis resulting in optic atrophy and blindness

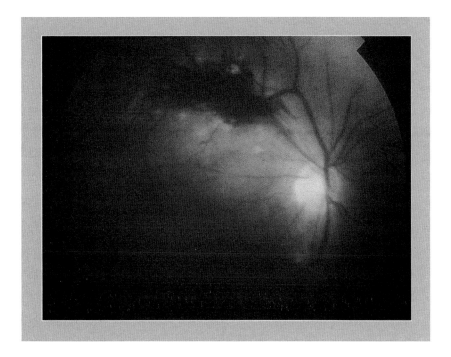

Figure 7.6   *Hemorrhagic CMV retinitis* A hemorrhagic lesion of CMV retinitis extending along the superior temporal vessels. This appearance is typically seen in more central CMV lesions

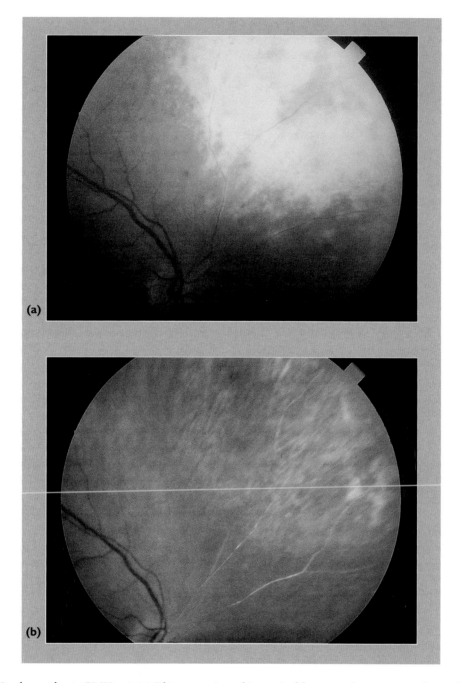

Figure 7.7   *Non-hemorrhagic CMV retinitis* This extensive white retinal lesion in the superonasal peripheral retina was only visible when the patient was asked to look up and to the left. The patient had no visual symptoms and the lesion was found on routine examination. Peripheral retinal lesions frequently have an agranular appearance with few hemorrhages. **(b)** After treatment, the whitened retina was replaced by an atrophic scar containing white, sclerosed, blood vessels. There is no difference in the rates of progression between hemorrhagic and non-hemorrhagic forms of CMV retinitis

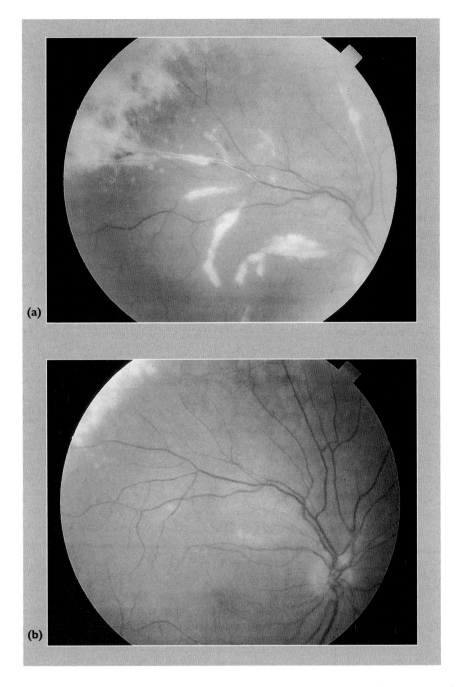

Figure 7.8   *Frosted-branch angiitis* **(a)** The macular blood vessels are obliterated by white perivascular inflammation. This appearance has given rise to the term 'frosted-branch angiitis'. The vascular sheathing (seen superiorly) represents an inflammatory reaction and is distinct from the retinal necrotic lesion caused by direct CMV infection. Inflammatory vasculitis, which has a similar appearance, has previously been described in immunocompetent patients. In HIV infection, it is seen in association with peripheral CMV retinitis. **(b)** The same patient as in (a). The result of treatment with intravenous ganciclovir is shown. There was rapid resolution of the vascular sheathing, but the peripheral lesion persisted and ultimately formed an atrophic scar

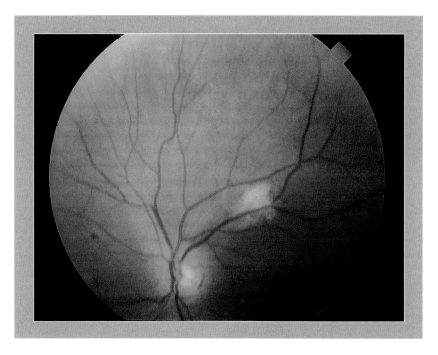

Figure 7.9   *CMV retinitis mimicking ocular toxoplasmosis* Fundoscopy shows an isolated focus of CMV retinitis along the superior temporal arcade with no associated hemorrhage This presents a similar appearance to that found in toxoplasmosis chorioretinitis or a fungal lesion

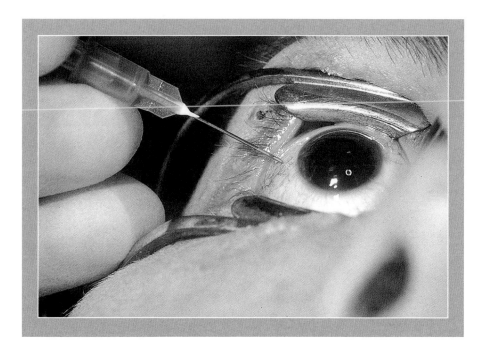

Figure 7.10   *CMV retinitis mimicking ocular toxoplasmosis – vitreal tap* When diagnostic uncertainty is present, a vitreal tap can be useful. Here the sample is analyzed using nucleic acid amplification techniques such as polymerase chain reaction for herpes viruses (CMV, varicella zoster virus, herpes simplex virus, etc.) as well as toxoplasmosis

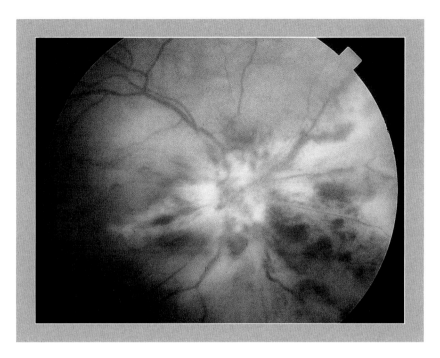

Figure 7.11 *CMV retinitis mimicking central retinal vein occlusion* Fundoscopy shows the optic disc obliterated by hemorrhage and necrotic retinal axons. The peripheral lesion nasal to the disc had expanded so that its active border reaches the optic disc

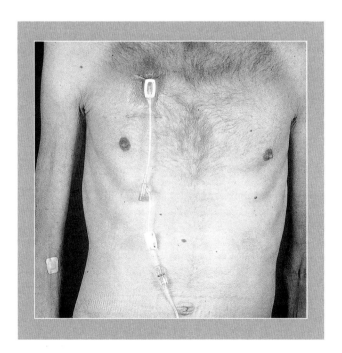

Figure 7.12 *Intravenous maintenance therapy* This is an example of the systems developed and widely used pre-HAART for CMV-maintenance therapy. A cannula sits within the reservoir of the totally implantable venous access central line (Port-A-Cath). The reservoir has been surgically placed under the skin of the chest. A flexible catheter runs under the skin, over the clavicle and into the internal jugular vein. The technique was designed for home administration. Apart from the side-effects of the drugs themselves, the disadvantages of the system included the disfiguring indwelling reservoir under the chest wall and the risk of infection from repeated needling (although the risk is less than that with Hickman lines). Treatment of CMV retinitis halts disease progression in up to 90% of cases, and is now often largely oral rather than intravenous therapy. If HAART is unavailable, prophylactic maintenance prolongs the duration of 'cure', but does not abolish the risk of relapse. Treatment must therefore be continued indefinitely

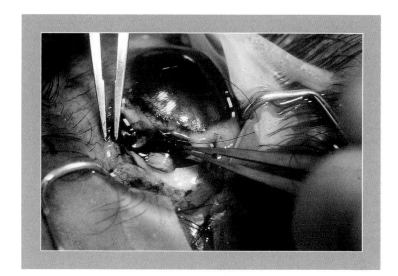

Figure 7.13 *Vitrasert sustained-release ganciclovir implant* This treatment device contains 4.5 mg of ganciclovir which passively diffuses into the vitreous cavity for 5–8 months. It is surgically implanted through a pars plana incision placed 4 mm from the limbus. The implant is anchored by a suture to the sclera. The short operation is performed under local anesthesia. Further implants may be inserted over time. Although these are an attractive option for local disease control, implants provided no protection against CMV infection outside the implanted eye. Risk factors for the development of bilateral retinitis include persistent fever, weight loss, previous AIDS diagnoses and positive CMV blood culture

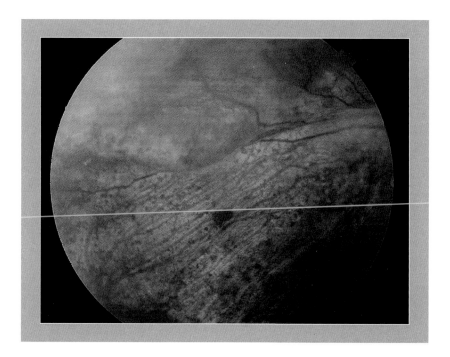

Figure 7.14 *Retinal detachment* Ten to twenty-five per cent of patients with CMV retinitis, develop detached retinas with a devastating loss of vision. Fundoscopy taken 1 year after the diagnosis of CMV retinitis, which scarred the macula and left the patient blind, shows the retinal CMV scar in the lower half of the field in sharp focus, whereas the upper half of the retina is detached forward and is thus indistinct. The superior blood vessels leaving the optic disc appear to bend as they are lifted forward together with the detached retina. Fluid has gained access to the subretinal space through the holes in the necrotic retina of the CMV scar and has separated the neurosensory retina from the pigment epithelium.

Retinal detachment may occur at any time after the diagnosis of CMV retinitis, although reports suggest that the risk increases with time from diagnosis and is typically seen with large peripheral lesions. This has important implications for treatment as both central and peripheral CMV may, therefore, lead to acute sight-threatening disease. As HAART prolongs survival, so the risk of retinal detachment has risen. It is now 60% by 12 months in patients who develop CMV disease. Retinal detachment in CMV retinitis is usually repaired by silicone oil tamponade after vitrectomy. Unfortunately, the current results with this procedure are far from satisfactory, and patients are often left with poor vision after surgical repair. There is also an increased risk of cataracts

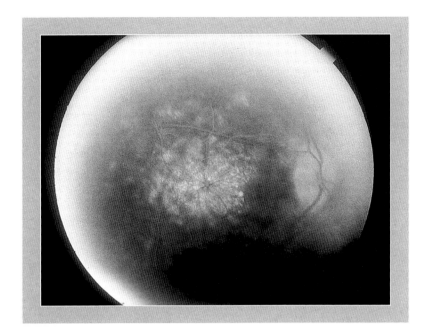

Figure 7.15 *Cystoid macular edema* Many inflammatory conditions give rise to an increase in the permeability of the parafoveal capillaries, resulting in cystoid macular edema. Essentially, fluid collects in the outer plexiform and inner nuclear layers of the retina and, as seen in this late-stage fluorescence angiogram, a petaloid pattern of hyperfluorescence appears as the dye fills the intraretinal spaces. The patient in this case had been treated for asymptomatic CMV retinitis for 1 year when he noticed a deterioration of visual acuity. The CMV retinitis was inactive and, on examination of the macula with a fundal lens, cystoid macular edema was observed. The common causes include cataract surgery, retinal vein occlusion, diabetic retinopathy and chronic uveitis. HAART has been reported to precipitate this condition, although almost 50% of cases are idiopathic

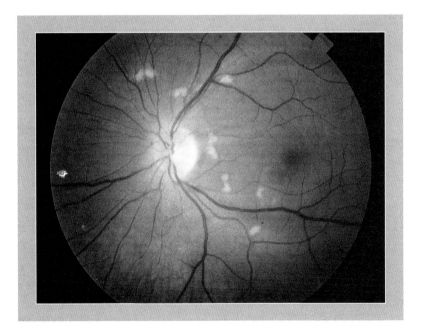

Figure 7.16 *HIV retinopathy* Routine fundoscopic examination of a patient with a CD4 count $< 50 \times 10^6/l$ revealed white fluffy foci scattered across the central retina. Their indented surface is typical of cotton wool spots. The patient had no visual symptoms and the lesions resolved spontaneously. Cotton wool spots are part of the microvasculopathy that occurs in response to retinal ischemia and are due to swelling of the nerve fiber layer. They produce no visual symptoms and tend to occur in the debilitated patient. Problems may arise in differentiating between an isolated cotton wool spot and an early focus of CMV retinitis

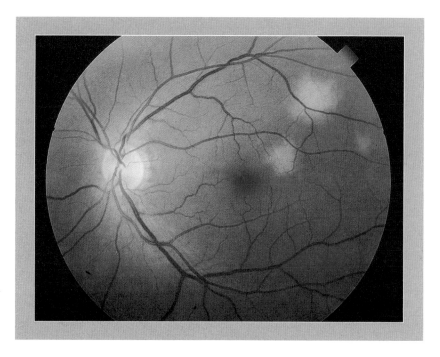

Figure 7.17 *Pneumocystis jiroveci choroiditis* The retinal features in this fundus are clearly visible as there is no vitreal inflammation. The discrete creamy-yellow, rounded, deep, choroidal lesions have the typical appearance of *Pneumocystis jiroveci* choroidopathy. The lesions regressed after specific antipneumocystis treatment. The patient had a previous history of PCP (*Pneumocystis* pneumonia) and had received inhaled pentamidine as secondary prophylaxis. However, this form of maintenance therapy does not protect extrapulmonary sites from recurrent disease

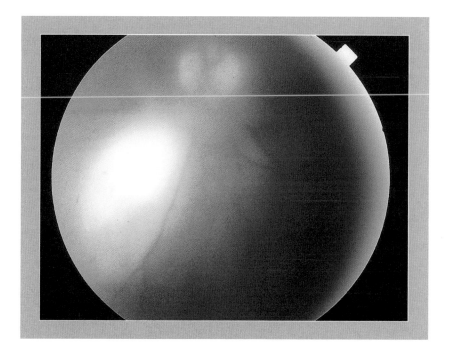

Figure 7.18 *Toxoplasmosis retinochoroiditis* The retina is hazy because of inflammatory cells within the vitreous. The optic disc is only barely distinguishable. Inferior to the disc is an oval-shaped white lesion of necrotizing retinochoroiditis. This appearance is described as 'headlights in the fog' and is due to a moderate vitritis which produces indistinct views of a single focus of retinal necrosis. The infection has newly disseminated to the eye. This is unlike reactivation of healed congenital *Toxoplasma gondii* scars seen in immunocompetent patients. Fifty per cent of HIV-infected individuals with retinal infection will have concurrent active cerebral toxoplasmosis

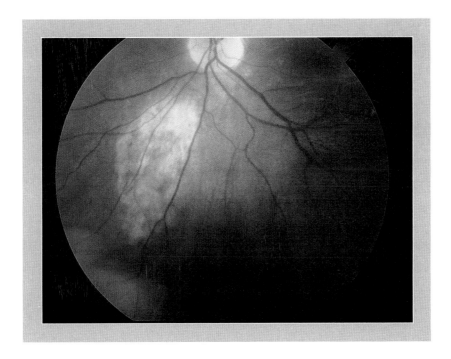

Figure 7.19 *Toxoplasmosis retinochoroiditis – inactive retinal scar* The patient's response to therapy was good with complete visual recovery. He was left with an inactive retinal scar

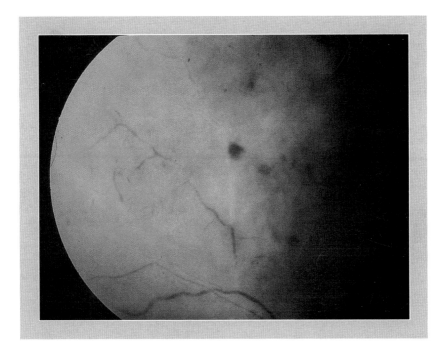

Figure 7.20 *Acute retinal necrosis* The peripheral retina superior to the macular blood vessels is pale, and contains blot hemorrhages and disrupted blood vessels due to full-thickness retinal necrosis. This had progressed over a 3-week period and resulted in a painless loss of vision. In immunocompetent patients, it is presumed to be due to herpes viral infections, and often has an associated large vessel vasculitis. HIV appears to promote more small vessel disease, and it may be seen with co-existent encephalopathy. In this case, vitreal PCR was negative for herpes simplex virus, CMV and varicella zoster virus, but positive for Epstein–Barr virus

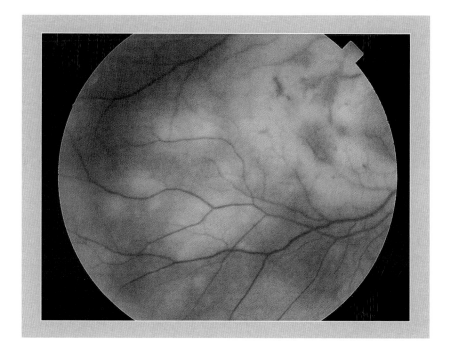

Figure 7.21 *Outer retinal necrosis* Fundoscopy shows extensive whitening of the deep (outer) retina which extends over the entire macula. The superficial retinal blood vessels course over the area and are apparently unaffected, hence the name of this disease. The condition is presumed to be caused by varicella zoster virus and, in up to 75% there is a history of shingles or other extra-ocular disease. It typically presents with a rapid loss of vision over a 24-h period

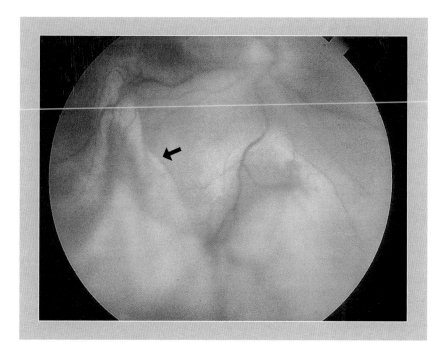

Figure 7.22 *Untreated outer retinal necrosis resulting in retinal detachment* The detached retina is seen as a thin white sheet billowing fowards and elevating the blood vessels. Subretinal fluid has separated the sensory from the retinal pigment epithelium. The sensory retina can be repositioned with surgically introduced silicone oil. However, when macular necrosis has occurred (as in this case), no improvement in vision will be gained with this procedure

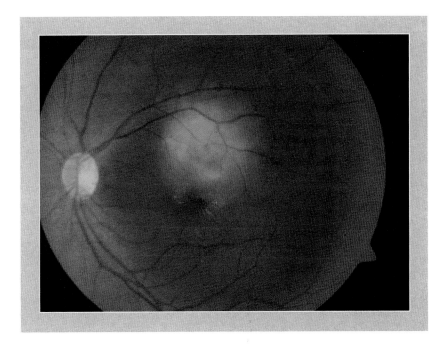

Figure 7.23 *Choroidal tuberculomata* This African patient had pulmonary tuberculosis and complained of blurred vision. Her left eye visual acuity was 6/36. The retinal photograph shows a raised, yellow, circumscribed mass of about two disc diameters in size at the posterior pole. The surrounding neurosensory retina is elevated and intraretinal exudates, in the form of a macular star, are visible. This large solitary mass has the typical appearance of a choroidal tuberculomata, which is present in 5% of cases of systemic tuberculosis. They are pathologically similar to tubercles found elsewhere in the body

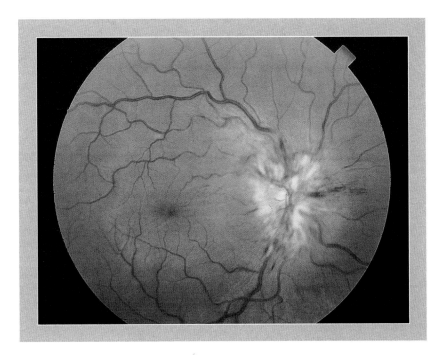

Figure 7.24 *Cryptococcal meningitis* Fundoscopy from a patient who complained of headache and blurred vision prior to admission to hospital, which was precipitated by a grand mal seizure. Lumbar puncture revealed *Cryptococcus* fungal infection and a high CSF opening pressure. *Cryptococcus* may also invade the optic nerve, causing papillitis. The optic disc seen here is enlarged and swollen. The blood vessels are dilated and tortuous, and there are circumferential retinal folds. Examination of the patient's visual field revealed an enlarged blind spot. There is established papilledema. This is present in up to 25% of cases of cryptococcal meningitis

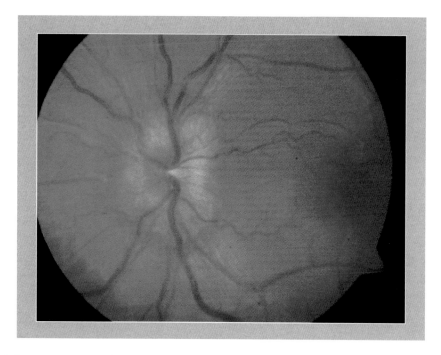

Figure 7.25   *Syphilitic optic neuritis* This left optic disc has blurred margins and is swollen. On examination, the patient had a visual acuity of 6/6 in both eyes but on visual field testing he had an enlarged left blind spot. A left relative afferent pupillary defect was present. Cranial nerve examination was otherwise normal and he had no signs of meningism. The CSF opening pressure was normal. He had a typical maculopapular skin rash of secondary syphilis. He complained of left ocular pain and blurred vision. This is the characteristic presentation of syphilitic optic neuritis, and should prompt exclusion of neurosyphilis by CSF examination. A swollen optic disc in secondary syphilis may also be caused by meningitis with papilledema

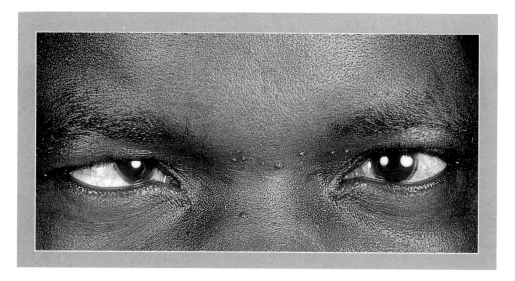

Figure 7.26   *Left sixth nerve palsy* This patient complained of double vision on looking to the left as illustrated. The paralysis of his left lateral rectus muscle arose from a sixth nerve palsy secondary to cerebral toxoplasmosis

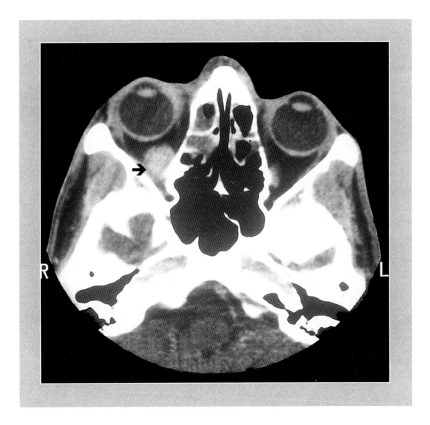

Figure 7.27   *Orbital mass* This enhanced axial CT scan of the orbits shows a discrete non-cavitating soft tissue intracranial mass at the apex of the right orbit (arrow). There is minor opacification in the right ethmoidal labyrinth as well as thickening of the soft tissue of the right globe

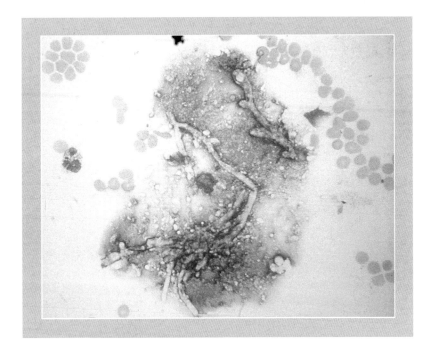

Figure 7.28   *Needle aspiration of orbital mass* Needle aspiration of the orbital mass in Figure 7.26 was performed. Romanowsky staining (MGG stain) revealed the dichotomously branching, septate hyphae, approximately 5 mm in diameter, of *Aspergillus*

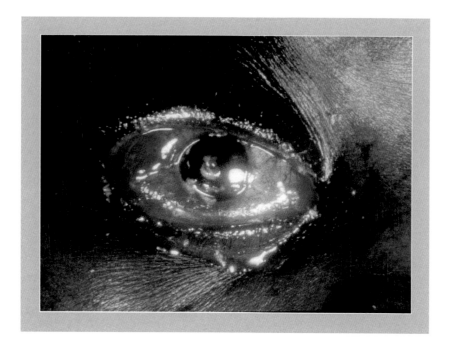

Figure 7.29 *Orbital reactive hyperplasia (pseudotumor)* This African patient's left eye is proptosed and the eyelids are blackened. The conjunctiva is inflamed and thickened with a diffuse mass. She presented with a severe follicular conjunctivitis which progressively became more painful over the next 2 weeks, and resulted in a painful proptosis. An incision biopsy of the periorbital mass showed chronic inflammation and no evidence for malignancy or infection. The reactive hyperplasia responded to radiotherapy. Conditions such as these are rare and probably reflect local chronic immune stimulation with subsequent mononuclear cell tissue infiltration

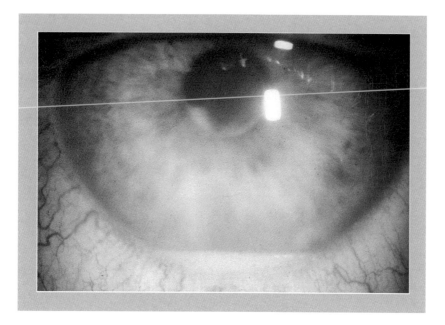

Figure 7.30 *Hypopyon uveitis* This patient, who had been treated for CMV retinitis, developed sudden loss of vision and a painful red eye. There is circumcorneal injection and the iris appears to be hazy due to inflammatory cells in the anterior chamber. These have settled to form a hypopyon, with a fibrinous exudate coating the lens at the pupillary margin. The inflammatory reaction was a consequence of drug therapy. The patient was taking both rifabutin and clarithromycin (which boosted the rifabutin to supranormal levels) for *Mycobacterium avium intracellulare* complex infection. On stopping the drugs, the uveitis spontaneously resolved. This has been reported in approximately 2–10% of early series when the drugs were used together. Rifabutin dose reduction has largely abolished this phenomenon. The presence of anterior uveitis should prompt a thorough examination of the eye and exclusion of retinal disease as well as syphilis

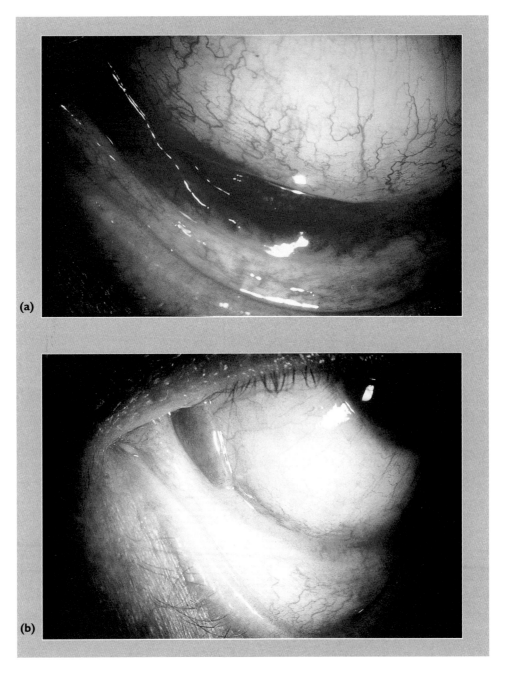

Figure 7.31 *Conjunctival Kaposi's sarcoma* This patient presented with a painless red eye. On examination of the inferior fornix, a discrete, violaceous, subconjunctival mass was seen **(a)**. This is the most common site of presentation of conjunctival Kaposi's sarcoma. The lesion regressed **(b)** as a result of the chemotherapy he was taking for the Kaposi's sarcoma present at other body sites

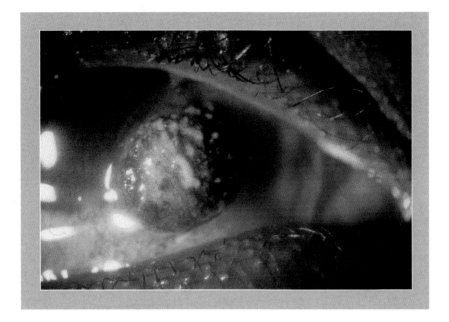

Figure 7.32 *Conjunctival squamous cell carcinoma* The illustration reveals recurrence of a conjunctival squamous cell carcinoma in the interpalpebral fissure in an African patient's right eye. The lesion is deeply pigmented, well-demarcated and round with an elevated uneven surface. There are white leukoplakia spots. It caused considerable discomfort and the conjunctiva was injected. The patient first presented with bilateral, interpalpebral, pigmented phlycten which were long-standing. In the right eye, the lesion enlarged and caused irritation. It was surgically removed, followed by a course of topical mitomycin chemotherapy. The lesion remained quiescent for 6 months before it recurred. The incidence of conjunctival squamous cell carcinoma in Africa increased with the epidemic of HIV. Exposure to ultraviolet light and papillomavirus have been implicated as co-factors

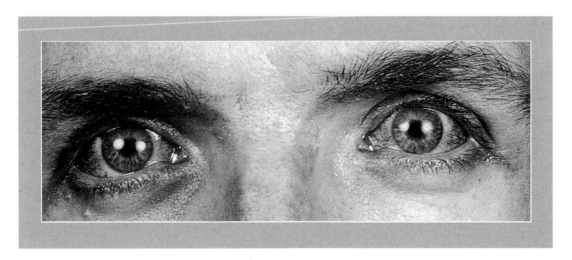

Figure 7.33 *HIV-related conjunctivitis* This patient complained of itchy red eyes and no visual loss. He presented with bilateral conjunctival hyperemia with a watery discharge. This was suggestive of a viral conjunctivitis but, as is often the case, swabs for viral and bacterial cultures were negative. CMV conjunctivitis has been described in HIV patients, but is rare. Other conditions that should be considered include microsporidial disease and conjunctival microvasculopathy. The theoretical increased risk of infections with either contact lens wearing or vision correction surgery (e.g. LASIK) has not been borne out in clinical practice

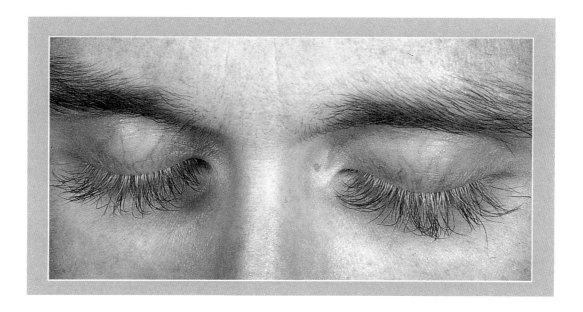

Figure 7.34 *Trichomegaly in HIV infection* This patient was HIV-positive, but did not have an AIDS diagnosis. He noted an increase in the length of his eyelashes. This feature has been reported at all stages of HIV infection and may arise from HIV-associated metabolic derangements. Outside HIV, trichomegaly is a recognized feature of both malabsorption and anorexia nervosa

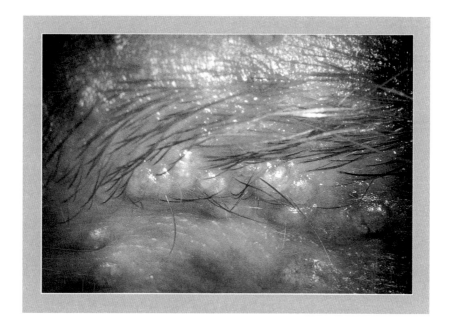

Figure 7.35 *Molluscum contagiosum* This is a poxvirus infection. The lesions may be either umbilicated or present a mosaic-like surface pattern. They are often multiple and can grow to up to 1 cm in size. Mollusca occur more commonly, and are less amenable to treatment, in patients with HIV infection. When they arise on the margin of the eyelid, the poxvirus may lead to conjunctivitis. In such cases, curettage of the lesions reduces the risk of further conjunctival disease

8

Malignant disease

The immune dysregulation associated with HIV increases the incidence of malignant disease. Kaposi's sarcoma and non-Hodgkin's lymphoma have a clear and consistent epidemiological association. For example, non-Hodgkin's lymphoma is 60 times more common than in the general population. Apart from these tumors, the incidence of all other cancers remained largely constant over the first decade of the HIV epidemic. Recently, there has been some evidence of an increased number of non-AIDS-defining malignancies, such as carcinoma of the lip, lung, cervix, penis, anus and Hodgkin's lymphoma. This is not supported by all studies, although it is certainly possible that the combination of lifestyle factors (e.g. smoking) together with the moderate degree of immunosuppression that probably still exists despite HAART in many patients, may increase the incidence of these tumors compared to HIV-negative individuals. Malignancies occur less frequently in children than in adults, although there is an excess of lymphoid tumors when compared to HIV-uninfected peers. Just as with both Kaposi's sarcoma and adult non-Hodgkin's lymphoma, this is in part driven by a viral co-pathogen. Kaposi's sarcoma is associated with HHV-8 infection, also known as Kaposi's sarcoma-associated herpes virus (KSHV). Children and adults who develop lymphoma can have high levels of circulating Epstein–Barr virus (EBV).

KAPOSI'S SARCOMA

Kaposi's sarcoma was the first tumor to be recognized as HIV-related and, initially, was seen in 40–50% of all AIDS cases. Recently, this has declined to 10%. This is not fully explained by the marked variation in its incidence within different HIV-positive risk groups (homosexual US males 20%, Caucasian US females 1%). It is also common in Africa, where, prior to HIV, an endemic form existed. KSHV has been demonstrated in all global variants of Kaposi's sarcoma.

Unlike the relatively benign 'classical' Kaposi's sarcoma seen in elderly, middle-European males, HIV-related Kaposi's sarcoma has a variable clinical picture. This ranges from 'benign' single lesions to aggressive, fatal multicentric visceral disease involving the lungs, gastrointestinal tract and lymph nodes.

Kaposi's sarcoma can regress on HAART. However, radiotherapy or chemotherapy may be indicated, if there is little response or extensive disease. There is some evidence that protease inhibitors have a direct anti-Kaposi's sarcoma effect, distinct from their potent antiretroviral activity.

NON-HODGKIN'S LYMPHOMA

Non-Hodgkins lymphoma is the second most common malignancy, accounting for at least 13% of all HIV-related tumors. It is usually an aggressive intermediate or high-grade B-cell type. There is a very strong association with EBV infection, which is oncogenic in this setting. This tumor has two forms: primary central nervous system (PCNS) and systemic non-Hodgkin's lymphoma. HAART has reduced the overall incidence of non-Hodgkin's lymphoma by approximately 40% – largely due to a reduction in PCNS type. The data are less clear for systemic non-Hodgkin's lymphoma, and it was estimated pre-HAART that, at 3 years from AIDS diagnosis, up to 40% of all patients would develop this tumor.

Systemic non-Hodgkin's lymphoma usually presents with marked constitutional symptoms, e.g. fever, night sweats and weight loss. The disease site is often extranodal (80% of cases) and typically includes the gastrointestinal tract, bone marrow and liver.

CNS lymphoma accounts for about 2% of all HIV-related malignancies. It presents as a solitary or multiple space-occupying lesion, responds poorly to any current therapy and has a median survival of 2 months. This malignancy is found late in HIV infection (CD4 $< 50 \times 10^6$/l). Systemic non-Hodgkin's lymphoma may present much earlier, and one-third of cases will have CD4 counts $> 200 \times 10^6$/l at diagnosis.

HODGKIN'S DISEASE

HIV infection may alter the clinical course of other malignancies, for example, Hodgkin's disease and papilloma virus-associated neoplasms. The rate of development of hepatocellular carcinoma in patients with cirrhosis is also increased due to a more rapid progression to end-stage liver disease. Hodgkin's disease occurs with a frequency eight times that of the general population. Patients tend to present with advanced disease and, consequently, the outcome is worse than for seronegative Hodgkin's disease patients. Prognosis correlates with CD4 count. HIV patients generally tolerate chemotherapy rather less well than the immunocompetent. This may be improved by granulocyte colony-stimulating factor (GCSF) or granulocyte–macrophage colony-stimulating factor (GM-CSF).

CERVICAL AND ANORECTAL CANCER

Cohort studies have suggested that there is an increased incidence of papilloma virus-associated anogenital neoplasia. As a result, the Centers for Disease Control (CDC) added invasive cervical cancer to the surveillance case definition of AIDS on the basis of aggressive clinical behavior when it occurs in HIV-infected women. The presence of cervical and anal intraepithelial neoplasia (CIN and AIN, respectively) are associated with each other and also with declining CD4 counts. Regular cervical smears, and possibly anal smears/biopsies, should be routine investigations among HIV-positive patients. HAART appears to have little effect on the natural history of either CIN or AIN. However, it is clear that these tumors will often spontaneously regress by themselves, making current cohort studies harder to interpret.

LUNG CANCER

The incidence of bronchogenic carcinoma may be increased in HIV infection. This occurs almost exclusively in smokers. Such individuals tend to be younger: patients are often less than 50 years old. Non-small carcinomas predominate, although, unlike the general population, adenocarcinoma is the most common histological subtype. There is some limited evidence that HIV-infected patients tend to progress more rapidly.

Despite these differences, the clinical presentation of lung cancer is similar in all populations. Symptoms include cough, breathlessness, chest pain, hemoptysis, malaise and weight loss. Typical radiographic findings include mediastinal adenopathy, hilar masses, parenchymal pulmonary tumors and pleural effusions. The differential diagnosis includes HIV-related opportunistic infections, Kaposi's sarcoma and non-Hodgkin's lymphoma.

TESTICULAR CANCER AND GERM CELL TUMORS

A high incidence of testicular cancer has been reported among HIV-positive individuals. Germ cell cancer is the most common malignancy in men under 40, the age below which HIV infection typically occurs in the developed world. It is, therefore, not surprising that several series have described germ cell cancers in a number of men with, or at risk of, HIV infection. Such malignancies have no recognized association with immunodeficiency. There may, however, be an increased incidence of seminoma in HIV-infected men compared with a control population.

Tumors in HIV-infected individuals are often treated with standard therapy according to their stage and histology. There is a high incidence of side-effects, although this is related to the patient's performance status. Systemic chemotherapy will, in general, reduce an individual's CD4 count by 50%. The use of HAART, as well as infection prophylaxis, is thus an important component of care.

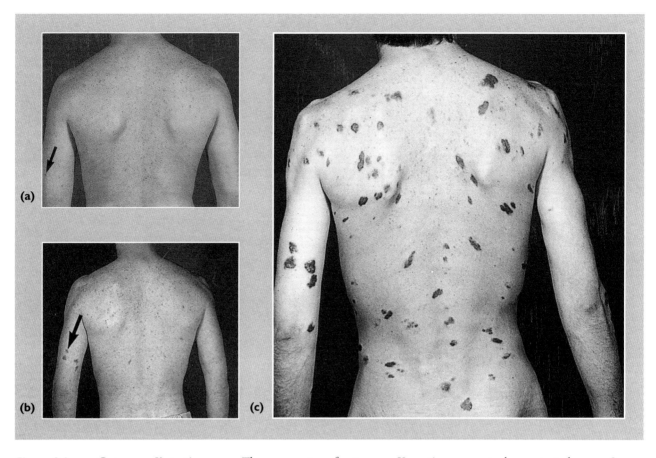

Figure 8.1 *Cutaneous Kaposi's sarcoma* The progression of cutaneous Kaposi's sarcoma is demonstrated over a 2-year period. Note the small purple lesions on the patient's left upper arm **(a)**, which slowly grow over 12 months **(b)**. New skin lesions start to appear symmetrically and line up along the skin creases between months 12 and 24 **(c)**. The patient shows features of marked weight loss, particularly muscle bulk and he died from pulmonary Kaposi's sarcoma at month 28. The risk of developing either of the most common HIV-related tumors, Kaposi's sarcoma or non-Hodgkin's lymphoma, increases by 40–50% with every $100 \times 10^6/l$ cell fall in blood CD4 count

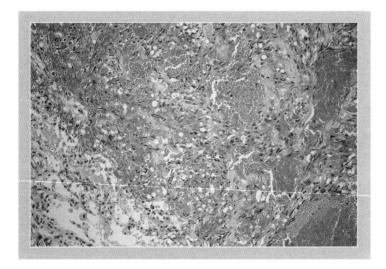

Figure 8.2 *Kaposi's sarcoma (H&E stain)* The lung is infiltrated by Kaposi's sarcoma. Spindle cells and extravasated red cells are seen to occupy most of the field. Distorted alveoli remain in the bottom left of the illustration. Kaposi's sarcoma derives from vascular or lymphatic endothelial cells. The demonstration that Kaposi's sarcoma-associated herpes virus (KSHV) is crucial in cell proliferation and tumor development has many implications for treatment and prevention. The virus appears to be transmissible in saliva, as well as sexually. It is likely that KSHV load in blood and oral fluids may predict the risk of future Kaposi's sarcoma, and thus be used to monitor high-risk individuals. HIV may further drive this process via cytokine and Tat protein production from HIV-infected cells

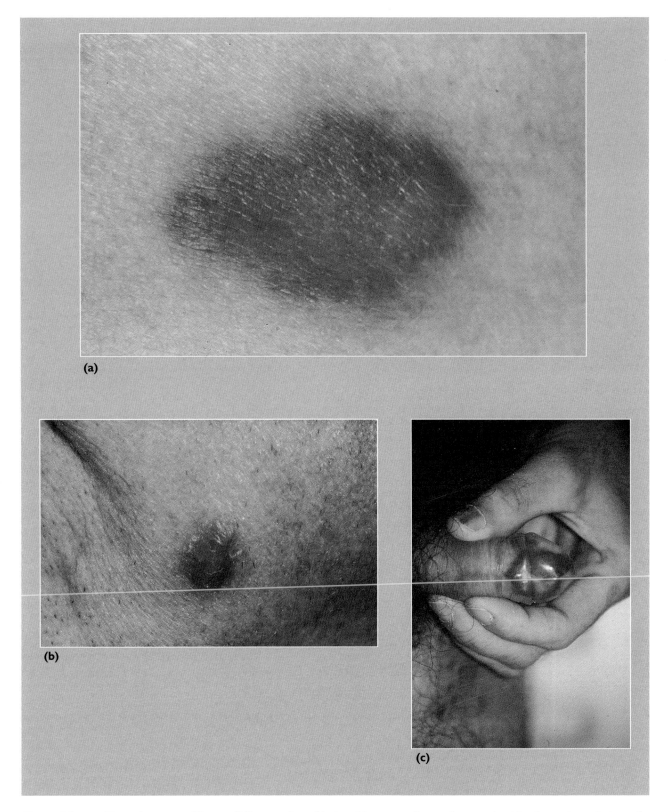

Figure 8.3   *Kaposi's sarcoma* The small flat purple-red lesion **(a)** was painless and not noticed by the patient. In its early stages, the tumor can be difficult to distinguish from a bruise and skin lesions such as this can be observed over a period of time. If doubt remains then biopsy is indicated. **(b)** A more advanced nodular Kaposi's sarcoma on the same patient's chin 6 months later. The rate at which the tumor progresses is variable. Kaposi's sarcoma on the face or genitals **(c)** can be cosmetically and psychologically damaging. Camouflage make-up can be as important as local therapy in managing these lesions, if HAART has not been effective

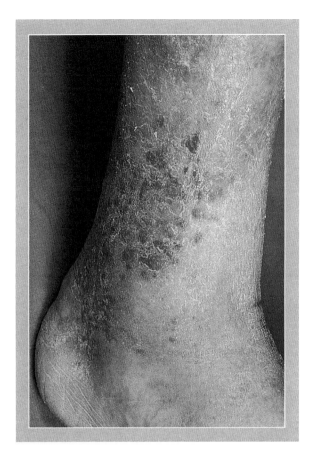

Figure 8.4 *Indurated Kaposi's sarcoma on the ankle* The Kaposi's sarcoma on this ankle has infiltrated subcutaneously producing a brawny indurated area

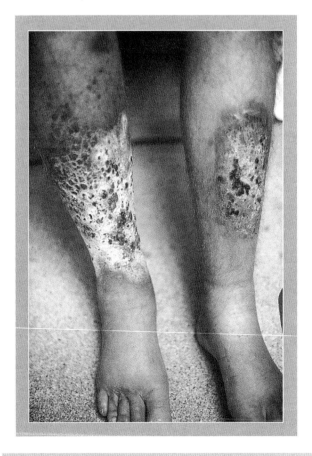

Figure 8.5 *Bilateral shin Kaposi's sarcoma* The extensive plaques of Kaposi's sarcoma have started to break down producing pain and pedal edema. This aggressive form of Kaposi's sarcoma can erode underlying tissues and bone

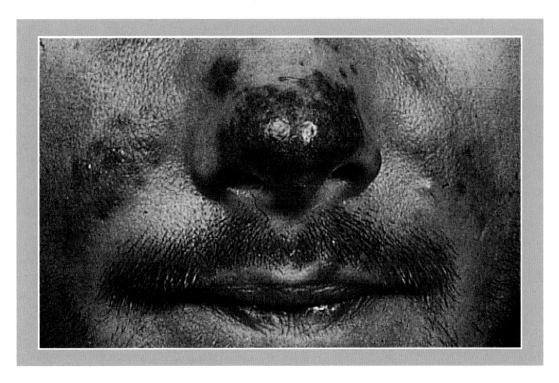

Figure 8.6   *Facial Kaposi's sarcoma* There is widespread Kaposi's sarcoma involving the nose, cheeks and lower lids. The marked facial edema is commonly seen in Kaposi's sarcoma and reflects lymphatic obstruction. Note also the widening of the bridge of the nose due to maxillary sinus involvement

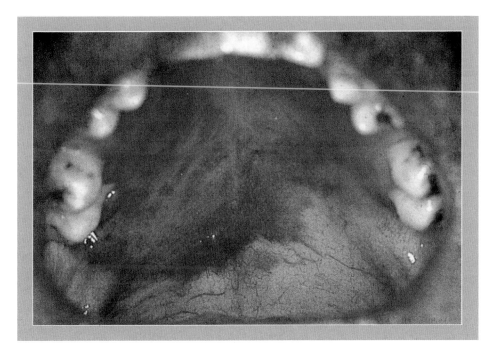

Figure 8.7   *Palatal Kaposi's sarcoma* Extensive disease involving most of the hard palate and gingiva. The patient was otherwise well and presented when his CD4 count was > 700 x 10^6/l. The lesion had only grown slowly over 18 months (for further examples see Chapter 4)

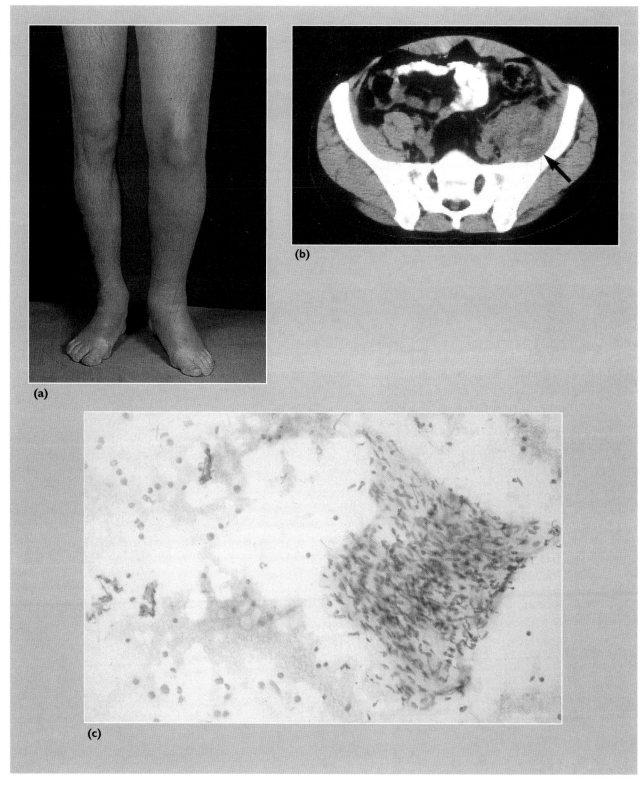

Figure 8.8   *Visceral Kaposi's sarcoma* The patient presented with back pain and a swollen left leg **(a)**. CT of the pelvis revealed an enlarged left iliopsoas muscle **(b,** arrow**)**. Percutaneous CT-guided needle biopsy demonstrated Kaposi's sarcoma. Cytology is a useful diagnostic technique in patients with visceral or nodal disease. The fine-needle lymph node aspirate **(c)** shows rafts of bland spindle cells consistent with Kaposi's sarcoma

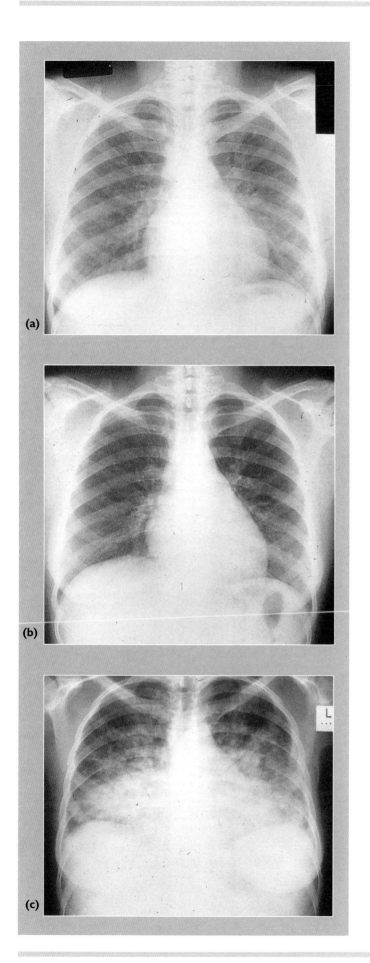

Figure 8.9 *Pulmonary Kaposi's sarcoma* The radiographs illustrate pulmonary Kaposi's sarcoma in an African woman with cutaneous Kaposi's sarcoma presenting with shortness of breath and hemoptysis. At month 0 **(a)** she had widespread reticulonodular shadowing but no hilar lymphadenopathy or pleural effusions. After 1 month of systemic chemotherapy, her symptoms and her chest radiograph had markedly improved **(b)**. Recurrence of breathlessness at month 9 was associated with extensive confluent shadowing and volume loss **(c)**. She died of respiratory failure 1 week after this radiograph was taken. Pulmonary Kaposi's sarcoma is typically reported in patients with very low CD4 counts ($< 50 \times 10^6$/l). It is associated with a poor prognosis from the onset of symptoms (median survival 9 months pre-HAART). There is some recent evidence that chemotherapy may improve the survival of what was managed previously with palliative care. Poor prognostic factors include older age and pleural involvement

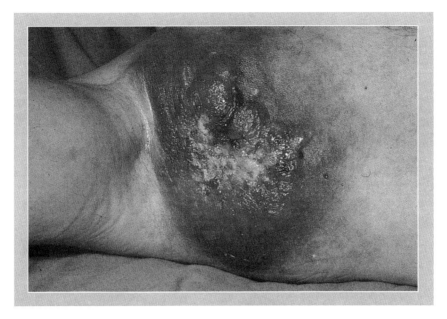

Figure 8.10 *Axillary lymphoma* The mass of axillary nodes enlarged rapidly and ulcerated. There were no other sites of disease. Histology demonstrated high-grade Burkitt's type non-Hodgkin's lymphoma which is seen in 30% of AIDS non-Hodgkin's lymphoma. The remainder are large cell (immunoblastic or large non-cleaved cell) lymphomas. Latent Epstein–Barr virus (EBV) infection and *c-myc* oncogene rearrangements are associated with the development of non-Hodgkin's lymphoma. However, the EBV genome can only be detected in 60% of large-cell lymphomas and 30% of the Burkitt's type. Kaposi's sarcoma-associated herpes virus (KSHV) is the causative agent of the rare primary effusion lymphoma (characterized by the presence of lymphomatous effusions in serosal cavities without solid masses), and Castleman's disease (angiofollicular lymphoid hyperplasia) in its multicentric form. The latter is often seen in the context of marked constitutional illness and even a sepsis-like syndrome. There are reports of Castleman's (not itself a clonal proliferation) evolving into plasmablastic lymphoma. This may be a cytokine-driven phenomenon as this condition is associated with very high levels of IL-6

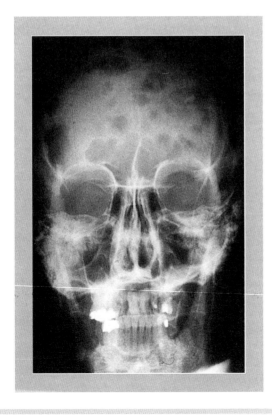

Figure 8.11 *Lymphomatous bony infiltration* The skull radiograph shows widespread, multiple, large lytic lesions in a man previously treated for abdominal non-Hodgkin's lymphoma. Lymphomas may recur in extranodal sites other than those initially involved. Asymptomatic leptomeningeal involvement is found in about 10% of patients. Lumbar puncture and CSF examination should be routinely performed when staging the tumors. Non-Hodgkin's lymphoma presenting as a first AIDS illness in patients with relatively well-preserved immune function (i.e. CD4 $> 150 \times 10^6$/l) responds to treatment. If chemotherapy is combined with HAART, median survival can be measured in years. Non-Hodgkin's lymphoma found in more advanced HIV disease or associated with CNS or bone marrow involvement (25% of cases at presentation), carries a worse prognosis with a median survival of months

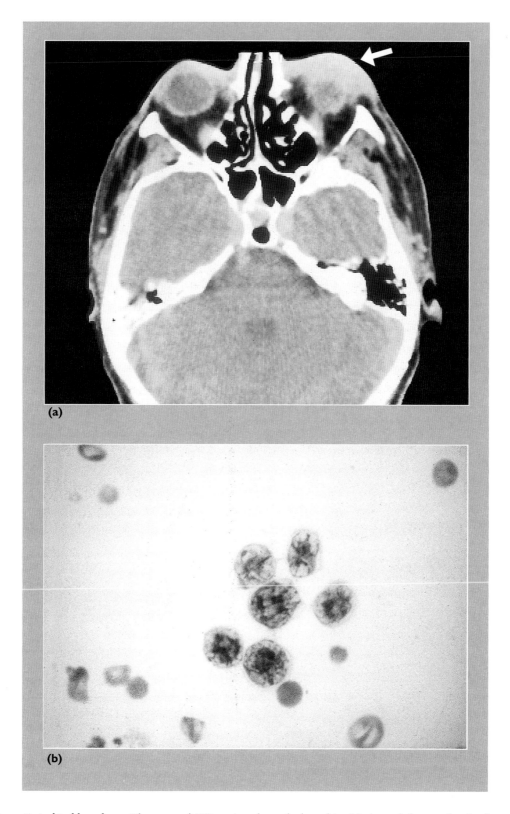

(a)

(b)

Figure 8.12 *Periorbital lymphoma* The coronal CT section through the orbits **(a)** shows left periorbital soft tissue swelling (arrow). This was associated with an enlarging left testis, right axillary lymphadenopathy and jaundice. Aspiration cytology of the periorbital lesion revealed high-grade B-cell non-Hodgkin's lymphoma **(b)**. High-grade tumors are often chemosensitive. Useful palliation may be achieved in late-stage disease with low-dose cytotoxic therapy

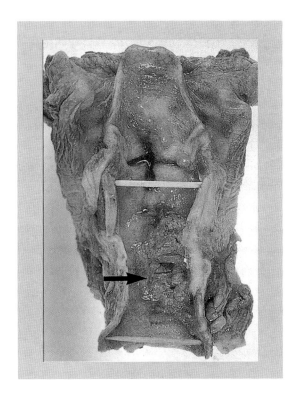

Figure 8.13 *Extranodal lymphoma* The tumor extending from a deposit in the thyroid ulcerated the anterior wall of the trachea (arrow). The patient presented with stridor rapidly progressing to obstruction and respiratory arrest. He was otherwise well, and his death resulted from the extranodal anatomical location rather than the extent of lymphomatous disease

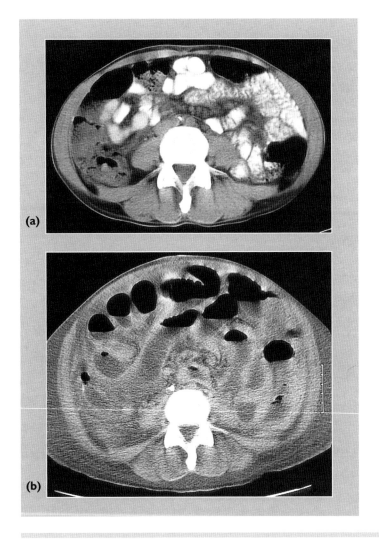

Figure 8.14 *Abdominal lymphoma* A 45-year-old HIV-infected male was investigated for non-specific but persistent periumbilical pain. A CT scan **(a)** revealed no abnormality. Over the next 4 months his pain became more frequent and he developed fevers, malaise and weight loss. He presented at month 4 of his illness with gross abdominal distension and bowel obstruction. A CT of the abdomen at this time **(b)** showed multiple thickened dilated loops of the small bowel. At laparotomy, he had encasement of his intestine with multiple dense adhesions. Biopsy confirmed non-Hodgkin's B-cell lymphoma. Despite palliative chemotherapy and infection prophylaxis, he died rapidly from sepsis

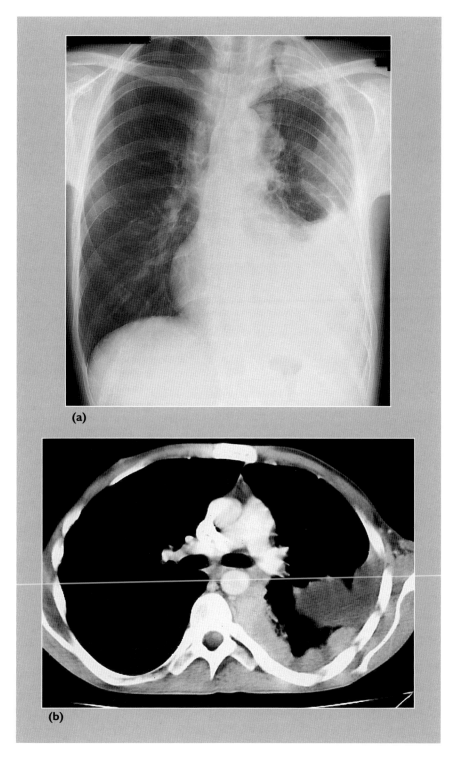

(a)

(b)

Figure 8.15 *Pleural adenocarcinoma* A 25-year-old male smoker presented with left-sided chest pain and breathlessness. The chest radiograph **(a)** shows lobulated pleural thickening extending down over the mediastinal surface, associated with pleural fluid. Aspiration cytology of the fluid revealed adenocarcinoma. The CT scan **(b)** confirms the extent of pleural involvement with extension along the oblique fissure. Although some debate exists over the frequency of HIV-related lung cancer, it does appear that HIV-positive smokers are at an increased risk of developing predominantly peripheral non-small-cell lung cancers at an earlier age. Sputum or pleural fluid cytology, histological and cytological evaluation of samples, obtained via bronchoscopy or by percutaneous fine-needle aspiration, are the most frequently used way of establishing the diagnosis. The outlook for this condition tends to be poor, despite aggressive management, including HAART and chemotherapy or surgery

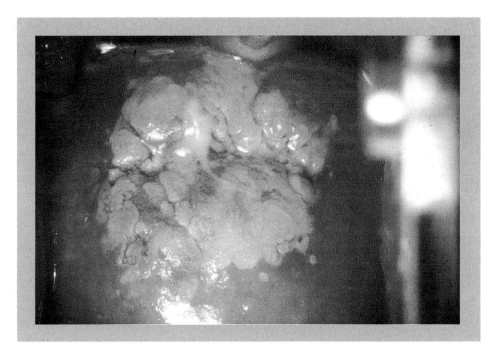

Figure 8.16 *Cervical intraepithelial neoplasia* A colposcopic view of the cervix after application of 5% acetic acid is shown. There are prominent aceto-white areas with a mosaic pattern indicating cervical intraepithelial neoplasia (CIN). The lesion was treated by local ablative therapy. Thirty per cent of HIV-positive women appear to have CIN. The incidence increases with advancing immunosuppression. It is frequently associated with perianal involvement (AIN). This has a similar prevalence to CIN, which is approximately three times greater than in the general population.

HIV-related CIN may be missed by smear testing alone. It appears to present at a later stage and is probably more rapidly progressive in women with low CD4 counts. As HAART does not appear to control either CIN or AIN it would be expected that there will be an increasing prevalence of HIV-related cervical and anal carcinoma. The latter will also be seen in males irrespective of their route of acquisition of HIV

9

HAART-related disease

The management of patients with HIV is a specialist area and should be performed by experts with appropriate experience and training. Treatment failure resulting from poor medication prescribing is an avoidable disaster. The mainstay of care is sensible decision-making and considered therapy. It is hoped that soon HAART will be available on a genuinely global basis. In the developed world, approximately two-thirds of HIV-infected patients are on medication. Quite apart from the regular monitoring that this entails, there is evidence that HIV survival and outlook depend upon the experience of the treating physician.

New drugs are in continuous development. As resistance to individual agents, and, more seriously, to classes of drugs develop, so the pressure to find further antiretroviral targets increases.

Drug development has been a remarkable collaboration between pharmaceutical companies, patients and clinicians. In many cases, production and licensing of drugs has been accelerated to enable promising chemicals to be tested more rapidly. This has led to the introduction of new agents which require careful post-marketing surveillance to monitor for side-effects.

The new class of fusion inhibitors have recently become licensed, while other novel agents, such as AXD-455 which blocks the release of RNA from the nucleus, are undergoing evaluation. If successful, this would open up a badly needed new target for therapeutic intervention.

The complexities of treatment cannot be overstated. New therapies continue to become available and licensed, and new data relating to existing medications render previous advice obsolete.

As experience with antiretroviral therapy has grown, and patients have been exposed to a wider range of agents over a prolonged period of time, it is apparent that HAART has unwanted side-effects. These are of varying severity and can be acute or of a chronic, insidious nature. In general, patients with advanced HIV tend to have more serious complications from treatment. Children tolerate medication reasonably well, although there are inevitably issues of adherence to complex regimens.

Side-effects from HAART involve a number of mechanisms. As with any drug, toxicity may arise from hypersensitivity. This can cause rashes, hepatic dysfunction, bone marrow suppression and a wide range of common side-effects – listed in Figure 9.1. Individual antiretroviral drugs demonstrate a number of idiosyncratic reactions, also outlined in Figure 9.1. The side-effects in children are similar in general to those seen in adults.

HAART seems to have a further property, however. Many of them, particularly nucleoside reverse transcriptase inhibitors (NRTIs) and possibly protease inhibitors, appear specifically to damage mitochondrial DNA, via inhibition of DNA polymerase-γ. This process would seem to be irreversible, and may be responsible for many of the syndromes associated with HAART, including lipodystrophy, hepatic steatosis, insulin resistance and pancreatitis. These features are also discussed in Chapter 5.

Abbreviations	Common name	Brand name	Common adverse reactions	Potential for interactions

Nucleoside reverse transcriptase inhibitors or nucleoside analogs (NRTIs)
Hepatotoxicity, mitochondrial toxicity/lactic acidosis with NRTIs

Abbreviations	Common name	Brand name	Common adverse reactions	Potential for interactions
AZT, ZDV	zidovudine	Retrovir	anemia, neutropenia, headaches, nausea, insomnia	minimal except for other marrow toxic medications
ddI	didanosine	Videx	diarrhea (buffered formulations), pancreatitis, peripheral neuropathy	buffered formulations: significant with medications whose absorption is decreased by buffers
ddC	zalcitabine	Hivid	peripheral neuropathy, oral ulcers	minimal except for other medications with neuropathic effects
d4T	stavudine	Zerit	peripheral neuropathy	minimal
3TC	lamivudine	Epivir	headaches, nausea	minimal
AZT/3TC		Combivir	same as AZT/3TC above	minimal
1592, ABC	abacavir	Ziagen	nausea, vomiting, diarrhea; hypersensitivity reaction (fever, malaise, gastrointestinal symptoms, rash, do NOT rechallenge)	minimal
AZT/3TC/ABC		Trizivir	same as AZT, 3TC, ABC above	minimal
FTC	emtricitabine	Emtriva, Coviracil	headache, diarrhea, nausea, rash, skin discoloration, lactic acidosis	minimal
ABC/3TC			same as ABC, 3TC above	minimal

Nucleotide reverse transcriptase inhibitors or nucleotide analogs
Increases in liver enzymes, lipase and bilirubin. Bone demineralization in animal studies

Abbreviations	Common name	Brand name	Common adverse reactions	Potential for interactions
(bis-POC) PMPA	tenofovir	Viread	nausea, vomiting, diarrhea and flatulence	Viread increases ddI levels by as much as 60%, increasing risk of pancreatitis and peripheral neuropathy. Possible interaction with nephrotoxic drugs (e.g. ganciclovir, aminoglycosides) relatively contraindicated with cidofovir as excretion pathways and drug interactions similar

Non-nucleoside reverse transcriptase inhibitors (NNRTIs)
Rash, hepatotoxicity with all NNRTIs

Abbreviations	Common name	Brand name	Common adverse reactions	Potential for interactions
NVP	nevirapine	Viramune	fatigue	both substrate and inducer of liver enzymes
DLV	delavirdine	Rescriptor	headache, fatigue	
EFV	efavirenz	Sustiva	CNS effects: dizziness, somnolence, insomnia, confusion	

Figure 9.1 *Antiretroviral drugs* Adverse reactions and interaction potential

Abbreviations	Common name	Brand name	Common adverse reactions	Potential for interactions
Protease inhibitors (PIs)				
Hepatotoxicity, lipodystrophy, dyslipidemias, insulin resistance/hyperglycemia with all PIs				
SQV	HGC-saquinavir	Invirase	diarrhea, nausea, abdominal pain	both substrate and inhibitor of liver enzymes
	SGC-saquinavir	Fortovase		
IDV	indinavir	Crixivan	nausea, raised bilirubin, kidney stones, dry skin and lips	both substrate and inhibitor of liver enzymes
RTV	ritonavir	Norvir	nausea, vomiting, diarrhea	SIGNIFICANT drug interactions due to potent inhibition of liver enzymes
NFV	nelfinavir	Viracept	diarrhea, nausea, vomiting	both substrate and inhibitor of liver enzymes
APV	amprenavir	Agenerase	nausea, diarrhea, rash, perioral/oral paraesthesias	both substrate and inhibitor of liver enzymes; formulated with vitamin E – AVOID Vitamin E supplements
ABT-378, LPV/r	lopinavir/ritonavir	Kaletra	diarrhea, nausea, cholesterol, trigylcerides, GGT	both substrate and inhibitor of liver enzymes; contains RTV, a potent inhibitor of liver enzymes
BMS-232632	atazanavir	Zrivada, Reyataz	hyperbilirubinemia, lipid abnormalities, hematuria cardiac disturbances	inhibitor of liver enzymes. Reduces efficacy of tenofovir, may lead to treatment failure. Reduces efficacy of efavirenz. Avoid lovastatin and simvastatin and St John's Wort
PNU-140690	tipranavir		diarrhea, nausea and stomach cramps. Vertigo, mood alterations, triglyceride elevations	reduces blood levels of delavirdine by 95%. Antacids, rifampicin reduce blood levels.
GW-433908	fos-amprenavir	Lexiva	nausea, vomiting, headache and rash	as amprenavir. May be combined with RTV, potent inhibitor of liver enzymes
Fusion inhibitors				
Local reactions at injection site				
T-20	enfuvirtide	Fuzeon	Pain and redness at injection site, headache, insomnia, peripheral neuropathy, eosinophilia	none yet documented

GGT, γ-glutamyltransferase

Figure 9.1 continued

HAART-associated lipodystrophy has been reported in both adults and children. It has a time-dependent course. Over the first 6 months of anti-retroviral therapy, there are increases in limb and central abdominal fat together with an increase in weight. However, progressive loss of limb fat occurs from then on (Figures 9.2 and 9.3). This is estimated to occur at a rate of 13% per year on HAART, and, with relatively limited follow-up, appears to be progressive. This lipoatrophy may be the key physical manifestation of lipodystrophy syndrome. Recent work has indicated that there appears to be little relationship between this and lipohypertrophy (e.g. an increase in visceral adipose tissue); and that the latter may in fact be no more common than in age-matched HIV-negative controls. Although this needs to be confirmed in large, prospective studies, it suggests that central fat accumulation is not a consequence of peripheral fat distribution.

Although all classes of anti-HIV drugs have been implicated, there are data to suggest that NRTIs, in particular stavudine, are particularly associated with lipoatrophy. Low baseline CD4 count (and subsequent maximal increase on HAART) appear to be linked to lipodystrophy. There is some evidence that protease inhibitors are more likely to cause a central abdominal fat type of lipohypertrophy (Figure 9.4). This may be associated with an increase in the dorsocervical fat (similar to the 'buffalo hump' of glucocorticoid excess; Figure 9.5).

The pathogenesis of lipodystrophy is poorly understood. What is clear is that normal adipocyte proliferation and differentiation do not occur in the presence of HAART. Instead of large, mature adipocytes the fat cells are small and irregular. The risk of lipodystrophy is increased in individuals with high baseline serum cholesterol levels. This presumably reflects already poorly functioning adipose tissue, and thus the addition of HAART further affects an already damaged system. This mechanism has been proposed for protease-related lipodystrophy. NRTIs inhibit DNA polymerase-γ which is required for mitochondrial DNA replication. This is thought to trigger events that lead to fat redistribution and, ultimately, fat loss.

Lipodystrophy can have a profound negative psychological impact on the individual. Changes in body shape are accompanied by a perception of aging, as well as a sense of 'reverting back' to the typical appearance of a patient with wasting and advanced HIV infection. This is particularly so for facial and buttock fat loss. In the latter case, the patient may also complain of pain on sitting (Figure 9.6). Figure 9.7 shows facial wasting. Note the prominent zygomatic arches with loss of both temporal and maxillary fat pads. The fat loss starts at the latter site and is evident on the 3-D laser scan which reproduces the topography of the face (Figure 9.8a). Treatments to improve this appearance include the use of subcutaneous injections of poly-lactic acid (NewFill®, Biotech Industries SA, Luxembourg). This stimulates collagen production under the skin without reducing dermal softness or elasticity. Most individuals require several treatments. The benefit is variable although in expert hands it is cosmetically satisfying, and sustained for months to years.

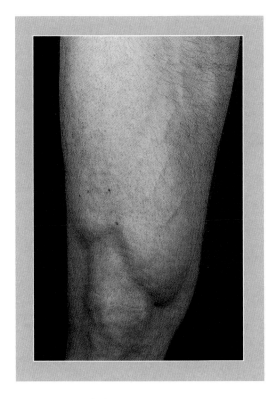

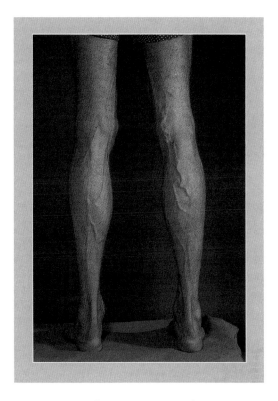

Figure 9.2   Limb fat wasting

Figure 9.3   *Leg fat wasting* Note the prominence of the superficial veins due to loss of the subcutaneous fat

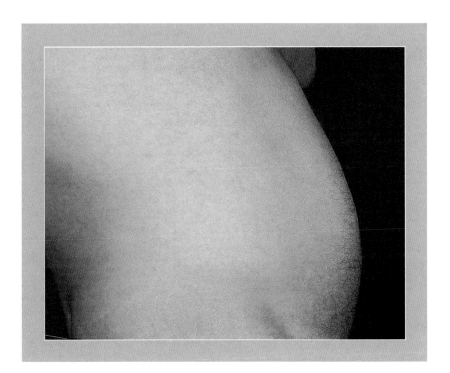

Figure 9.4   Visceral fat hypertrophy

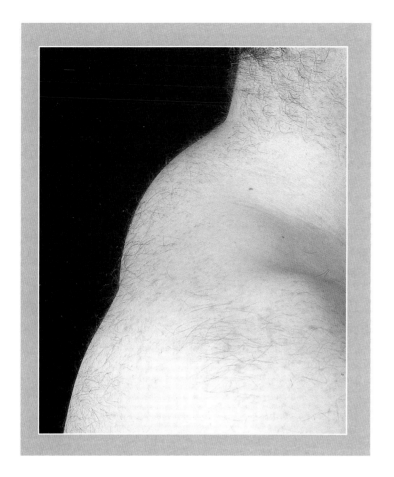

Figure 9.5 *Dorsocervical fat pad* The phenomena demonstrated here and in Figure 9.4 are associated with insulin resistance and possible subsequent development of diabetes and cardiovascular disease, the latter being via accelerated formation of atheromatous plaques in major arteries. It is important to pay attention to traditional risk factors for heart attacks and strokes such as smoking, hypertension and high alcohol consumption

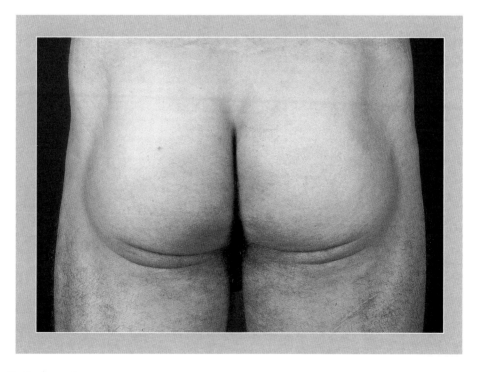

Figure 9.6 Buttock wasting

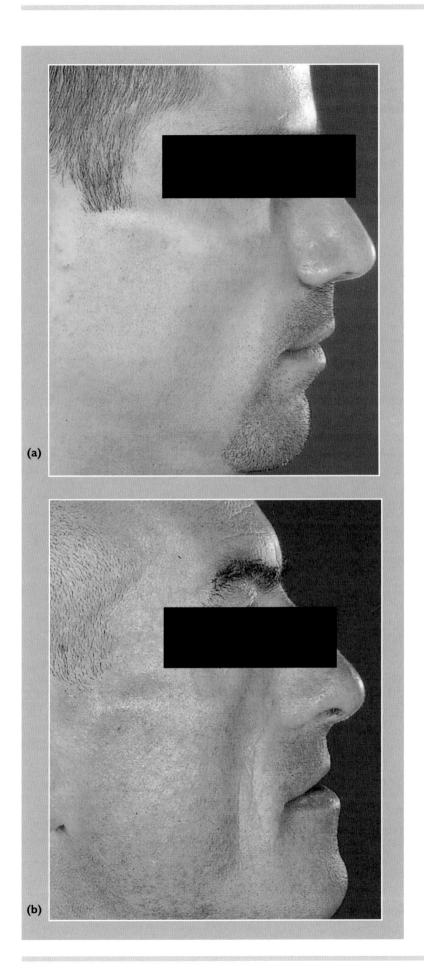

Figure 9.7   *Facial   wasting*   **(a)** Mild; **(b)** severe

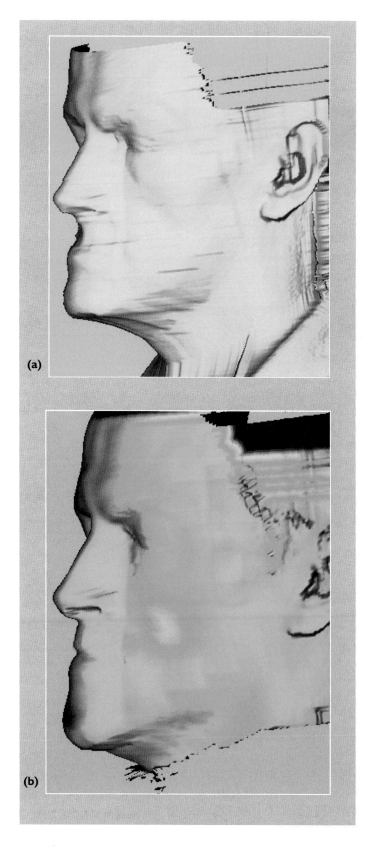

Figure 9.8   *Facial wasting* 3-D laser scans reproducing the topography of the face. **(a)** Loss of fat from the face is demonstrated. **(b)** The same patient is shown after a course of polylactic acid injections. The change from baseline is represented by colors ranging from yellow to green. The pretreatment sunken cheeks have largely disappeared

There are increasing reports of patients starting HAART who develop either new infection-related symptoms (e.g. CMV retinitis despite relatively high CD4 counts) or transient worsening of pre-existing disease. This immune restoration inflammatory syndrome (IRIS) is thought to reflect the restoration of pathogen-specific immune responses causing inflammation within tissues already infected by that pathogen. It typically occurs within days to weeks of starting HAART (Figure 9.9), and has been reported with mycobacteria (e.g. tuberculosis and MAC), viruses (e.g. herpes viruses, papilloma and polyoma virus, and hepatitis B and C) and fungi (e.g. cryptococcus and histoplasmosis). There are also reports implicating this phenomenon in viral-related diseases such as Kaposi's sarcoma (KSHV) and lymphoma (EBV).

Symptoms can last anywhere from a few months to more than 1 year. The distinction between infection and post-infectious inflammation can be difficult and sometimes patients will require treatment for both. IRIS can mimic drug reactions.

Immune-mediated illnesses may be prevented by starting anti-HIV treatments before CD4 counts drop below 200×10^6/l, although this may not be true in all illnesses, for example, tuberculosis.

Patients with mycobacterial disease seem especially prone to IRIS. The reported incidence varies widely, but probably about 25% of all patients with tuberculosis will have a transient deterioration in symptoms after starting HAART (the paradoxical reaction). This appears to be unrelated to the patient's starting blood CD4 count, although it is more frequently seen in patients who experience a rapid reduction in HIV load and those with disseminated tuberculosis. This might explain why it is much more common than in HIV-uninfected individuals (where it occurs in up to 10%). In the latter case, localized, single-site disease is the norm.

IRIS is almost always a clinical definition, as there is no definitive diagnostic test. In some cases, pathogens (both live and dead) can be recovered from the site of disease activity. Thus, it may be easily confused with pure immune deficiency-related illnesses. Pathological studies have focused on the host immune response (certain MHC haplotypes seem to predispose to IRIS, cytokine levels are different with or without IRIS). However, it is likely that the ability of a specific organism to elicit an immune response is also important. Specific relationships include TNF polymorphisms in MAC, while hepatitis C viral activity increases with rising CD4 counts. Recurrence of herpes zoster (shingles) correlates with a high initial rebound in levels of CD8 T cells.

There is no accepted treatment for IRIS, although this will often involve both anti-infectives and anti-inflammatories. There is rarely an indication to stop HAART, although treatment should be monitored closely for unwanted interactions. Support should be provided to enable the patient to continue on the various drug regimens prescribed during this time.

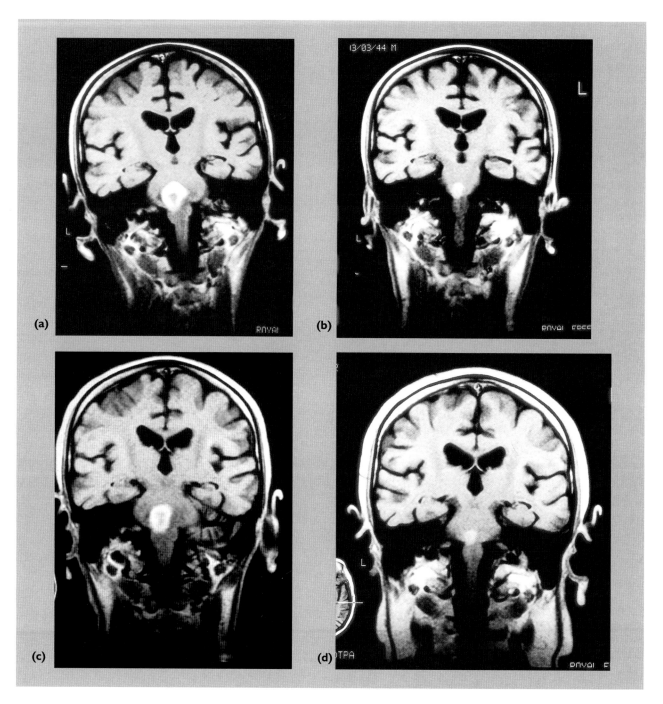

Figure 9.9 *Immune restoration inflammatory syndrome (IRIS)* The serial MRI scans are those of an individual who presented with pulmonary tuberculosis and was found to be HIV-infected. He was started on antituberculous treatment and his respiratory symptoms improved. His CD4 count was $60 \times 10^6/l$ and he began HAART after 3 weeks of antituberculous treatment. During week 2 of his antiretroviral therapy, he developed increasing confusion. The MRI scan of the brain **(a)**, reveals a space-occupying mass within the lower pons. This was associated with multiple cerebral lesions. The patient was started on corticosteroids and made a rapid recovery associated with an improvement in the scan appearance **(b)**. HAART and antituberculous medication were continued and the dose of steroids was gradually reduced. However, several weeks later (when he was taking prednisone 10 mg/day), he once more became confused and developed diplopia. The scan shown in **(c)**, obtained at this time, reveals recurrence of his pontine lesion. Re-institution of an increased dose of steroid resulted in symptomatic improvement and a follow-up MRI scan confirmed the associated reduction in CNS disease **(d)**. Despite extensive investigations no organisms were recovered from samples once he had started his tuberculosis medication. He completed this, but required a similar length of steroid treatment to prevent further 'paradoxical reactions' while on therapy

For unknown reasons skin reactions are more common in HIV infection, especially in late-stage disease. Almost all drugs can cause a rash in hypersensitive individuals although some are more common; up to one-sixth of patients on nevirapine will develop a rash. It may be more severe in about 2%. The frequency can be reduced if the drug is introduced at a half dose for the first 2 weeks. However, a skin reaction associated with abnormal liver function tests is an indication to discontinue the drug permanently. Rashes associated with abacavir may represent a hypersensitivity reaction in about 4% of cases. This can be fatal if the patient is rechallenged. If suspected (clinically the patient continues to deteriorate while on abacavir with fever, rash and possibly breathlessness or diarrhea), the individual should never receive the drug again.

Most neurological changes that occur with HAART are beneficial. In particular, the poor prognoses associated with PML and HIV encephalopathy have markedly improved with successful treatment.

Efavirenz is associated with transient neurological abnormalities, including sleep disturbance, nightmares and mood alteration. Some individuals find these symptoms so disturbing that they discontinue the medication. However, they tend to resolve after the first 4 weeks of treatment.

Drug-induced neuropathies can be very painful. Antiretroviral NRTIs such as stavudine, didanosine and zalcitabine may cause peripheral neuropathy. They can exacerbate otherwise minor neuropathies. Drug-induced symptoms are often, if variably, reversible with discontinuation or, preferably, dose reduction of the drug. Interactions may occur with other treatments, e.g. isoniazid in antituberculosis therapy, where up to 40% of individuals co-administered stavudine develop neuropathy. Another similar important drug interaction is with the chemotherapeutic agent vincristine used in the treatment of lymphoma and Kaposi's sarcoma.

Diarrhea is often associated with HAART. Common causes include protease inhibitors which produce increased gut motility. These include nelfinavir (up to 50% of patients), amprenavir, saquinavir and ritonavir. Antidiarrheal agents such as loperamide provide useful symptomatic relief. NRTIs such as didanosine, and abacavir can also lead to diarrhea.

A number of antiretrovirals are associated with acute, occasionally fatal, hemorrhagic pancreatitis. They are mostly the nucleoside analogs, particularly didanosine and stavudine. Less than 10% of patients taking didanosine will have biochemical evidence of pancreatitis, manifested as an increase in serum pancreatic amylase. Pentamidine and ganciclovir are also potent causes of pancreatitis.

Figure 9.10 *Ingrowing toenail* The protease inhibitor indinavir can cause ingrowing toenails, although this may be partly an HIV effect. The co-administration of NRTIs such as lamivudine has been implicated. Long-term treatment with AZT may cause blue-gray discoloration of the nails. The discoloration usually starts about 4–8 weeks after beginning the drug. Hydroxyurea has been reported to have a similar effect in black-skinned individuals. Indinavir also causes dry skin and hair loss. This is possibly via an effect on the major cell differentiation factor SREBP-1

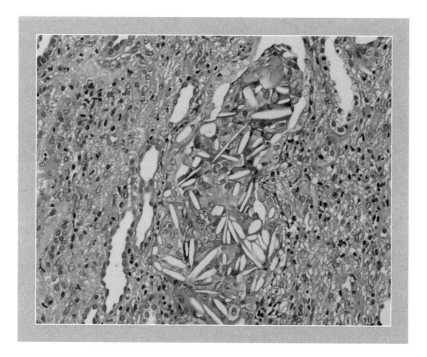

Figure 9.11 *Indinavir crystals* Long-term use of indinavir is associated with the development of renal stones as the drug precipitates within the kidney. The kidney biopsy (PAS stain) shows the needle- and rectangular-shaped crystals of indinavir within a tubular lumen associated with a macrophage reaction. There is a surrounding tubulo-interstitial nephritis within the renal parenchyma. The reported incidence of this condition is 4%. Recent work has suggested a much higher frequency than this (up to 30%). The lower figure may reflect the incidence of symptomatic disease, with acute renal colic and hematuria, while a much greater number of individuals will develop progressive renal dysfunction and subclinical kidney stone formation. Nephrolithiasis can be reduced by increasing daily fluid intake, although, on average, stones develop after approximately 5 months of treatment and are more common in older individuals. This group are probably at greater risk of progressive renal damage from such insults

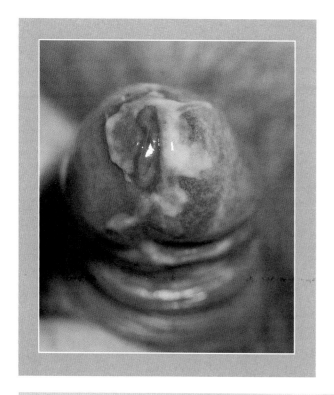

Figure 9.12 *Penile ulceration* The patient developed this condition while taking foscarnet. This drug has both some anti-HIV and CMV activity, although also frequently produces significant side-effects. The most common of these is renal impairment, seen in up to one-third of patients

Selected bibliography

HIV: AN OVERVIEW

Bowen EF, Sabin CA, Wilson P, *et al.* Cytomegalovirus (CMV) viraemia detected by polymerase chain reaction identifies a group of HIV-positive patients at high risk of CMV disease. *AIDS* 1997;11:889–93

Centers for Disease Control. 1993 Revised classification system for HIV infection and expanded surveillance case definition for AIDS among adolescents and adults. *Morb Mortal Wkly Rep* 1992;41:RR-17

DeSimone JA, Pomerantz RJ, Babinchak TJ. Inflammatory reactions in HIV-1-infected persons after initiation of highly active antiretroviral therapy. *Ann Intern Med* 2000;133:447–54

Dorrucci M, Rezza G, Vlahov D, *et al.* Clinical characteristics and prognostic value of acute retroviral syndrome among injecting drug users. *AIDS* 1995;9:597–604

Feldman JG, Gange SJ, Bacchetti P, *et al.* Serum albumin is a powerful predictor of survival among HIV-1 infected women. *J Acquir Immune Defic Syndr* 2003;33:66–73

Goulder PJ, Jeena P, Tudor-Willliams G, *et al.* Paediatric HIV infection: correlates of protective immunity and global perspectives in prevention and management. *Br Med Bull* 2001;58:89–108

Grossman Z, Meier-Schellersheim M, Sousa AE, *et al.* CD4+ T-cell depletion in HIV infection: are we closer to understanding the cause? *Nat Med* 2002;8:319–23

Hooper E. *The River: A Journey to the Origins of HIV and AIDS*. London: Penguin, 1999

Lederman MM, Valdez H. Immune restoration with anti-retroviral therapies: implications for clinical management. *J Am Med Assoc* 2000;284:223–8

Levy JA. HIV pathogenesis and long-term survival. *AIDS* 1993;7:1401–10

Luzuriaga K, Bryson Y, Krogstad P, *et al.* Combination treatment with zidovudine, didanosine, and nevirapine in infants with human immunodeficiency virus type 1 infection. *N Engl J Med* 1997;336:1343–9

McCune JM. The dynamics of CD4+ T-cell depletion in HIV disease. *Nature* 2001;410:974–9

Mertens TE, Hayes RJ, Smith PG, *et al.* Epidemiological methods to study the interaction between HIV infection and other sexually transmitted diseases. *AIDS* 1990;4:57–65

Michael NL, Moore JP. HIV-1 entry inhibitors: evading the issue. *Nat Med* 1999;5:740–1

Mocroft A, Ledergerber B, Katlama C, *et al.*; EuroSIDA Study Group. Decline in the AIDS and death rates in the EuroSIDA study: an observational study. *Lancet* 2003;362:22–9

Musey L, Hughes J, Schacker T, *et al.* Cytotoxic-T-cell responses, viral load, and disease progression in early human immunodeficiency virus type 1 infection. *N Engl J Med* 1997;337:1267–74

Newell ML. Prevention of mother-to-child transmission of HIV: challenges for the current decade. *Bull World Health Organ* 2001;79:1138–44

Pantaleo G, Graziosi C, Demarest JF, *et al*. HIV infection is active and progressive in lymphoid tissue during the clinically latent stage of disease. *Nature* 1993;362:355–8

Pantaleo G, Graziosi C, Fauci AS. New concepts in the immunopathogenesis of human immunodeficiency virus. *N Engl J Med* 1993;328:327–35

Pedersen C, Lindhardt BO, Jensent BL, *et al*. Clinical course of primary HIV infection: consequences for subsequent course of infection. *Br Med J* 1989;299:154–7

Philpott S, Burger H, Charbonneau T, *et al*. CCR5 genotype and resistance to vertical transmission of HIV-1. *J Acquir Immune Defic Syndr* 1999;21:189–93

Saif MW, Greenberg B. HIV and thrombosis: a review. *AIDS Patient Care STDs* 2001;15:15–24

Schacker T, Collier AC, Hughes J, *et al*. Clinical and epidemiologic features of primary HIV infection. *Ann Intern Med* 1996;125:257–64

Sinicco A, Fora R, Sciandra M, *et al*. Risk of developing AIDS after primary acute HIV1 infection. *J Acquir Immune Defic Syndr* 1993;6:575–81

van Rij RP, Portegies P, Hallaby T, *et al*. Reduced prevalence of the CCR5 delta32 heterozygous genotype in human immunodeficiency virus-infected individuals with AIDS dementia complex. *J Infect Dis* 1999;180:854–7

UNAIDS. *Gender and HIV*. Fact Sheet. Geneva: UNAIDS, 2001, August

UNAIDS. *Report of the Global HIV/AIDS Epidemic*. Geneva: UNAIDS, 2002, July

UNAIDS. *AIDS Epidemic Update*. Report. Geneva: UNAIDS, 2002, December

Zhu T, Mo H, Wang N, *et al*. Genotypic and phenotypic characterization of HIV-1 inpatients with primary infection. *Science* 1993;261:1179–81

SKIN DISEASE

Berger TG. Dermatologic care in the AIDS patient. In Sande MA, Volberding PA, eds. *The Medical Management of AIDS*, 5th edn. Philadelphia: W.B. Saunders Co., 1997

Buchbinder SP, Katz MH, Hessol NA, *et al*. Herpes zoster and human immunodeficiency virus infection. *J Infect Dis* 1992;166:1153–6

Gordin FM, Simon GL, Wofsy CB, *et al*. Adverse reactions to trimethoprim-sulfamethoxazole in patients with acquired immunodeficiency syndrome. *Ann Intern Med* 1984;100:492–8

Harris PS, Saag MS. Dermatologic manifestations of human immunodeficiency virus infection. *Curr Probl Dermatol* 1997;9:212–42

Manfredi R, Calza L, Chiodo F. Epidemiology and microbiology of cellulitis and bacterial soft tissue infection during HIV disease: a ten year survey. *J Cutan Pathol* 2002;29:168–72

Penneys NS. *Skin Manifestations of AIDS*, 2nd edn. London: Dunitz, 1995

Reynaud-Mendel B, Janier M, Gerbaka J, *et al*. Dermatologic findings in HIV-infected patients: a prospective study with emphasis on the CD4 count. *Dermatology* 1996;192:325–8

Rico MJ, Myers SA, Sanchez MR. Guidelines of care for dermatologic conditions in patients infected with HIV. Guidelines/Outcomes Committee. American Academy of Dermatology. *J Am Acad Dermatol* 1997;37:450–72

Rotunda A, Hirsch RJ, Scheinfeld N, *et al*. Severe cutaneous reactions associated with the use of human immunodeficiency virus medications. *Acta Derm Venereol* 2003;83:1–9

RESPIRATORY DISEASE

Badri M, Wilson D, Wood R. Effect of highly active antiretroviral therapy on incidence of tuberculosis in South Africa: a cohort study. *Lancet* 2002;359:2059–64

Burman WJ, Jones BE. Treatment of HIV-related tuberculosis in the era of effective antiretroviral therapy. *Am J Respir Crit Care Med* 2001;164:7–12

Castro M. Treatment and prophylaxis of *Pneumocystis carinii* pneumonia. *Semin Respir Inf* 1998;13:296–303

Diaz PT, Wewers MD, Pacht E, *et al.* Respiratory symptoms among HIV-seropositive individuals. *Chest* 2003;123:1977–82

Masur H, Kaplan JE, Holmes K; US Public Health Service; Infectious Diseases Society of America. Guidelines for preventing opportunistic infections among HIV-infected persons – 2002. Recommendations of the US Public Health Service and the Infectious Diseases Society of America. *Ann Intern Med* 2002;137:435–78

Mayaud C, Parrot A, Cadranel J. Pyogenic bacterial lower respiratory tract infections in human immunodeficiency virus-infected patients. *Eur Respir J Suppl* 2002;36:28s–39s

Miller RF. Prophylaxis of Pneumocystis carinii pneumonia: too much of a good thing? *Thorax* 2000;55(Suppl 1):S15–22

Phair J, Munoz A, Detels R, *et al.* The risk of *Pneumocystis carinii* pneumonia among men infected with human immunodeficiency virus type 1. *N Engl J Med* 1990;332:161–5

Rerkpattanapipat P, Wonpraparut N, Jacobs L, *et al.* Cardiac manifestations of acquired immunodeficiency syndrome. *Arch Intern Med* 2000;160:602–8

Sub-committee of the Joint Tuberculosis Committee of the British Thoracic Society. Management of opportunist mycobacterial infections: Joint Tuberculosis Committee guidelines 1999. *Thorax* 2000; 55:210–18

The Interdepartmental Working Group on Tuberculosis. UK guidance on the prevention and control of transmission of 1. HIV-related tuberculosis, and 2. Drug-resistant, including multiple drug-resistant tuberculosis. The prevention and control of tuberculosis in the United Kingdom. London: Department of Health, 1998, September

Zumla A, Johnson MA, Miller R, eds. *AIDS and Respiratory Medicine*. London: Chapman & Hall, 1997

GASTROINTESTINAL DISEASE

American Gastroenterological Association medical position statement: guidelines for the management of malnutrition and cachexia, chronic diarrhea, and hepatobiliary disease in patients with human immunodeficiency virus infection. *Gastroenterology* 1996;111:1722–3

British HIV Association HIV/hepatitis B and HIV/hepatitis C co-infection guidelines, 2003. http://www.bhiva.org/guidelines.htm

Cohen J, West AB, Bini EJ. Infectious diarrhea in human immunodeficiency virus. *Gastroenterol Clin North Am* 2001;30:637–64

Dieterich DT, Wilcox CM. Diagnosis and treatment of esophageal diseases associated with HIV infection. Practice Parameters Committee of the American College of Gastroenterology. *Am J Gastroenterol* 1996;91:2265–9

Greenspan JS, Barr CE, Sciubba JJ, *et al.* (USA Oral AIDS Collaborative Group). Oral manifestations of HIV infection. Definitions, diagnostic criteria and principles of therapy. *Oral Surg Oral Med Oral Pathol* 1992;73:142–4

Tedaldi EM, Baker RK, Moorman AC, *et al.* Influence of coinfection with hepatitis C virus on morbidity and mortality due to human immunodeficiency virus infection in the era of highly active antiretroviral therapy. *Clin Infect Dis* 2003;36:363–7

Weinert M, Grimes RM, Lynch DP. Oral manifestations of HIV infection. *Ann Intern Med* 1996;125:485–96

ENDOCRINE, METABOLIC, MUSCULO-SKELETAL AND RENAL DISEASE

Bhasin S, Singh AB, Javanbakht M. Neuroendocrine abnormalities associated with HIV infection. *Endocrinol Metab Clin North Am* 2001;30:749–64

Brown P, Crane L. Avascular necrosis of bone in patients with human immunodeficiency virus infection: report of 6 cases and review of the literature. *Clin Infect Dis* 2001;32:1221–6

Bureau NJ, Cardinal E. Imaging of musculoskeletal and spinal infections in AIDS. *Radiol Clin North Am* 2001;39:343–55

Chene G, Angelini E, Cotte L, *et al.* Role of long-term nucleoside-analogue therapy in lipodystrophy and metabolic disorders in human immunodeficiency virus-infected patients. *Clin Infect Dis* 2002;34:649–57

Dobs A, Brown T. Metabolic abnormalities in HIV disease and injection drug use. *J Acquir Immune Defic Syndr* 2002;31(Suppl 2):S70–7

HIV Lipodystrophy Case Definition Group. An objective case definition of lipodystrophy in HIV-infected adults: a case–control study. *Lancet* 2003;361:726–35

John M, Mallal S. Hyperlactatemia syndromes in people with HIV infection. *Curr Opinion Infect Dis* 2002;15:23–9

Kakuda TN. Pharmacology of nucleoside and nucleotide reverse transcriptase inhibitor-induced mitochondrial toxicity. *Clin Ther* 2000;22:685–708

Kimmel PL, Barisoni L, Kopp JB. Pathogenesis and treatment of HIV-associated renal diseases: lessons from clinical and animal studies, molecular pathologic correlations, and genetic investigations. *Ann Intern Med* 2003;139:214–26

Schambelan M, Benson CA, Carr A on behalf of the International AIDS Society-USA. Management of metabolic complications associated with antiretroviral therapy for HIV-1 infection: recommendations of an International AIDS Society-USA panel. *J Acquir Immune Defic Syndr* 2002;31:257–75

NEUROLOGICAL DISEASE

Anderson E, Zink W, Xiong H, *et al*. HIV-1-associated dementia: a metabolic encephalopathy perpetrated by virus-infected and immune-competent mononuclear phagocytes. *J Acquir Immune Defic Syndr* 2002;31(Suppl 2):S43–54

Cardoso F. HIV-related movement disorders: epidemiology, pathogenesis and management. *CNS Drugs* 2002;16:663–8

Clifford DB. AIDS dementia. *Med Clin North Am* 2002;86:537–50

Gisslen M, Hagberg L. Antiretroviral treatment of central nervous system HIV-1 infection: a review. *HIV Med* 2001;2:97–104

Schifitto G, McDermott MP, McArthur JC, *et al*.; Dana Consortium on the Therapy of HIV Dementia and Related Cognitive Disorders. Incidence of and risk factors for HIV-associated distal sensory polyneuropathy. *Neurology* 2002;58:1764–8

Simpson DM, Wolfe DE. Neuromuscular complications of HIV infection and its treatment. *AIDS* 1991;5:917–26

Skiest DJ. Focal neurological disease in patients with acquired immunodeficiency syndrome. *Clin Infect Dis* 2002;34:103-15

OCULAR DISEASE

Jabs DA. Ocular manifestations of HIV infection. *Trans Am Ophthalmol Soc* 1995;93:623–83

Jabs DA, Gilpin AM, Min YI, *et al*. Studies of Ocular Complications of AIDS Research Group. HIV and cytomegalovirus viral load and clinical outcomes in AIDS and cytomegalovirus retinitis patients: Monoclonal Antibody Cytomegalovirus Retinitis Trial. *AIDS* 2002;16:877–87

Jabs DA, Van Natta ML, Kempen JH, *et al*. Characteristics of patients with cytomegalovirus retinitis in the era of highly active antiretroviral therapy. *Am J Ophthalmol* 2002;133:48–61

Kestelyn PG, Cunningham ET Jr. HIV/AIDS and blindness. *Bull World Health Organ* 2001;79:208–13

Ormerod LD, Larkin JA, Margo CA, *et al*. Rapidly progressive herpetic retinal necrosis: a blinding disease characteristic of advanced AIDS. *Clin Infect Dis* 1998;26:34–45

Wright ME, Suzman DL, Csaky KG, *et al*. Extensive retinal neovascularization as a late finding in human immuno-deficiency virus-infected patients with immune recovery uveitis. *Clin Infect Dis* 2003;36:1063–6

MALIGNANT DISEASE

Bower M, Powles T, Nelson M, *et al*. HIV-related lung cancer in the era of highly active antiretroviral therapy. *AIDS* 2003;17:371–5

Cattelan AM, Trevenzoli M, Aversa SM. Recent advances in the treatment of AIDS-related Kaposi's sarcoma. *Am J Clin Dermatol* 2002;3:451–62

Chin-Hong PV, Palefsky JM. Natural history and clinical management of anal human papillomavirus disease in men and women infected with human immunodeficiency virus. *Clin Infect Dis* 2002;35:1127–34

Frisch M, Biggar RJ, Engels EA, Goedert JJ; AIDS-Cancer Match Registry Study Group. Association of cancer with AIDS-related immunosuppression in adults. *J Am Med Assoc* 2001;285:1736–45

Minkoff H, Ahdieh L, Massad LS, *et al*. The effect of highly active antiretroviral therapy on cervical cytologic changes associated with oncogenic HPV among HIV-infected women. *AIDS* 2001;15:2157–64

Pollock BH, Jenson HB, Leach CT, *et al*. Risk factors for pediatric human immunodeficiency virus-related malignancy. *J Am Med Assoc* 2003;289:2393–9

Stebbing J, Portsmouth S, Bower M. Insights into the molecular biology and sero-epidemiology of Kaposi's sarcoma. *Curr Opin Infect Dis* 2003;16:25–31

Vaccher E, Spina M, Tirelli U. Clinical aspects and management of Hodgkin's disease and other tumours in HIV-infected individuals. *Eur J Cancer* 2001;37:1306–15

HAART-RELATED DISEASE

Dieleman JP, van Rossum AM, Stricker BC, *et al*. Persistent leukocyturia and loss of renal function in a prospectively monitored cohort of HIV-infected patients treated with indinavir. *J Acquir Immune Defic Syndr* 2003;32:135–42

Fichtenbaum CJ, Gerber JG. Interactions between antiretroviral drugs and drugs used for the therapy of the metabolic complications encountered during HIV infection. *Clin Pharmacokinet* 2002;41:1195–211

Friis-Moller N, Weber R, Reiss P, *et al*. Cardiovascular disease risk factors in HIV patients – association with anti-retroviral therapy. Results from the DAD study. *AIDS* 2003;17:1179–93

Hadigan C, Meigs JB, Wilson PW, *et al*. Prediction of coronary heart disease risk in HIV-infected patients with fat redistribution. *Clin Infect Dis* 2003;36:909–16

Johnson AA, Ray AS, Hanes J, *et al*. Toxicity of antiviral nucleoside analogs and the human mitochondrial DNA polymerase. *J Biol Chem* 2001;276:40847–57

Kontorinis N, Dieterich DT. Toxicity of non-nucleoside analogue reverse transcriptase inhibitors. *Semin Liver Dis* 2003;23:173–82

Lichtenstein KA, Delaney KM, Armon C, *et al*. for the HIV Outpatient Study Investigators. Incidence of and risk factors for lipoatrophy (abnormal fat loss) in ambulatory HIV-1-infected patients. *J Acquir Immune Defic Syndr* 2003;32:48–56

Madge S, Kinloch-de-Loes S, Mercey D, *et al*. Lipodystrophy in patients naive to HIV protease inhibitors. *AIDS* 1999;13:735–7

Mallon PW, Miller J, Cooper DA, *et al*. Prospective evaluation of the effects of antiretroviral therapy on body composition in HIV-1-infected men starting therapy. *AIDS* 2003;17:971–9

Shelburne SA III, Hamill RJ. The immune reconstitution inflammatory syndrome. *AIDS Rev* 2003;5:67–79

van der Valk M, Reiss P. Lipid profiles associated with antiretroviral drug choices. *Curr Opin Infect Dis* 2003;16:19–23

White AJ. Mitochondrial toxicity and HIV therapy. *Sex Transm Infect* 2001;77:158–73

Index

investigations 19, 21
ischemic retinopathy 142
Isospora 38, 84, 98

jaundice 105
JC virus 135

Kaposi's sarcoma 39, 163, 166–171
    cutaneous 42, 59, 166, 167–169
    epidemiology 38
    gastrointestinal 93
    ocular 141, 161
    oral 83, 91, 169
    pulmonary 63, 79, 166, 171
    tracheal 80
    visceral 170
Kaposi's sarcoma-associated herpes virus (KSHV)
    59, 161, 164, 172
keratoderma blennorrhagica 44
kidney stones 186

lactic acidosis 113
leishmaniasis 94
libido, decline in 110
lichenoid drug reaction 57
linear gingival erythema 90
lipoatrophy 111
lipodystrophy 111–113, 180, 182
lipohypertrophy 111, 180, 182
liver disease 38, 84, 105–108, 115
    cirrhosis 106
liver function tests 105
long-term non-progressors 22
low-density lipoprotein (LDL) 111
lung biopsy 62
lung cancer 164
lung collapse 73
luteinizing hormone (LH) 110
lymphadenopathy 27, 29–31
    paraortic 94
    tuberculosis 65
lymphocytic interstitial pneumonitis (LIP) 77
lymphoma 42, 172–174
    abdominal 174
    axillary 172
    bony infiltration 172
    extradural 139
    extranodal 174
    gastrointestinal 93
    periorbital 173
    primary CNS lymphoma 121, 129–131, 163–164
    primary effusion 172
    see also non-Hodgkin's lymphoma
lymphomatous effusion 80

macrocytosis 33, 34
macular rash 41
    during seroconversion 26, 27

maternal–fetal transmission 11–12
mediastinal lymphadenopathy 29
membranous glomerulonephritis 118
meningitis 138
    cryptococcal 121, 138, 142, 156
    tuberculous 131
meningoencephalitis 26, 122
methadone 38
MHC molecules, gp120 homology with 16
Microsporidia 38, 84, 96, 98–99
miliary tuberculosis 66
mitochondrial toxicity 113, 117, 177
molluscum contagiosum 41, 46, 141, 160
mononeuritis complex 140
mononeuritis multiplex 123
mortality 9, 10, 20
    HAART impact 10, 20
mouth ulcers 41, 83, 88–90
    during seroconversion 26
    ulcerative gingivitis 90
    ulcerative periodontitis 90
multiple sclerosis 134
musculoskeletal disease 116–117
mycobacteria 94–95
Mycobacterium avium complex (MAC) 23, 26, 62,
    66, 99
    fever and 31
Mycobacterium tuberculosis 64, 66
    skin ulceration 51
    see also tuberculosis
Mycobacterium xenopi 67
myopathy 121

nail changes 41, 44, 45, 187
    ingrowing toenails 187
    zidovudine-induced 58
natural history of infection 20–26
    seroconversion 26–27, 28, 122
    variation in 22
necrotizing gingivitis 90
necrotizing periodontitis 90
needlestick injury 14
Neisseria meningitidis 138
nephrotic syndrome 117, 118
nevirapine 41, 56, 178, 187
Nikolsky's sign 57
Nocardia 63
non-Hodgkin's lymphoma 23, 80, 163–164
    cerebellar 131
    extradural 139
    gastrointestinal 93

onycholysis 44
onychomycosis 45
opportunistic infections 23, 26
    CNS infections 121
    developing world 38
    treatment 63

sexual behavior, transmission and 9–10
sexually transmitted infection 35–38
shingles 49
sinusitis 125
sixth nerve palsy 157
skin infections 41
    bacterial 49–52
    fungal 45
    protozoal 53
    viral 46–49
skin rashes 41
    drug-induced 56, 178–179
    during seroconversion 26
    papulopruritic eruptions 54, 57
smoking 79, 164
soft tissue disease 38, 39
spinal cord disease 138
splenic abscess 94
splenomegaly 94
sputum culture 62, 68, 69
squamous cell carcinoma, conjunctival 162
Staphylococcus aureus
    endocarditis 38
    pulmonary infection 72
    skin disease 41, 48, 49, 50
stavudine 113, 178
Stevens–Johnson syndrome 56, 57, 141
Streptococcus pneumoniae 63, 72, 73, 125, 138
Streptococcus pyogenes 49
Streptococcus viridans 38
strongyloidiasis 77
subacute inflammatory demyelinating neuropathy 123
subtypes of HIV 12–13
swallowing difficulties 83–84
syncytia formation 15–16
syphilis 35, 83
    membranous glomerulonephritis 118, 119
    ocular 142, 157

testicular cancer 164–165
testicular infection 110
testing *see* HIV antibody tests; HIV antigen tests
testosterone levels 109–111
thiacetazone 38
thrombocytopenia 33
thyroid disease 109
tinea capitis 45
tinea cruris 45
tinea pedis 45
toxic epidermal necrolysis 41, 57
toxoplasmosis 76
    CNS infections 121, 126–128, 157
    ocular infection 142
    prophylaxis 26
    retinochoroiditis 153–154
transmission 9–10
    prevention strategies 13
    risk to health-care workers 13–14

vertical transmission 11
trichomegaly 160
triglycerides 110, 111
tuberculoma 133
    choroidal 156
tuberculosis 31, 52, 61–62, 64–65
    cerebral abscess 133
    cerebral infarction 132
    chemoprophylaxis 62
    CNS lesions 121
    developing world 38
    lymphadenopathy 65
    meningitis 131
    miliary 66
    multidrug resistance 62
    ocular 140
    pericarditis 81
    therapy 61–62
tuberculosis granuloma 31, 32
ulceration
    duodenal 93
    during seroconversion 26, 31
    esophageal 84, 93
    genital 35, 48, 188
    mouth 27, 41, 83, 88–90
    mucosal 57
    perianal 102, 103
    skin 50, 51
ultrasensitive tests 18
urine tests 18
urticaria 41
uveitis 36, 141
    hypopyon 162
    immune recovery uveitis 142

vacuolar myelopathy 122, 138
vaginal *Candida* infection 37
varicella zoster *see* herpes zoster
vasculitis 59
vertical transmission 11
viral cultures 18
viral warts 36, 38, 41, 47
virology 14–16
vulval herpes 37

warts, viral 36, 38, 41, 47, 103
    genital 47
    perianal 103
wasting 38, 84, 95, 110, 180, 182–184
    facial 179, 183–184
Western blot 17–18

zalcitabine 178
zidovudine 41, 178
    blood disease and 33, 34
    mitochondrial toxicity 113, 117
    nail changes and 58